"Misdiagnosis is rampant in today's world. Maybe you don't have multiple sclerosis, maybe you don't have bladder problems, maybe you don't have arthritis, or chronic fatigue, or neuropathy... maybe it's your thyroid! So many are being treated for diseases they don't have. In today's world, you have to do your own research. The Women's Guide to Thyroid Health is the most informative, thorough guide to understanding the thyroid you will ever read. Discover why you are not feeling well. Kathryn Simpson has done the work; you will be the beneficiary. This is the best book explaining the thyroid that I have ever read."

—Suzanne Somers

"This book is an excellent overview of endocrine function in women, with particular emphasis on the importance of thyroid activity. The reader will be well informed of the critical interaction between multiple bodily functions and endocrine activity. A must-read for men and women who seem to be suffering the effects of 'normal' aging. A hormone adjustment may result in a more enjoyable and healthy life. This work can potentially be a true life-changer for thousands of Americans."

—Scot A. Brewster, MD, cardiac surgeon at Scripps Hospital in La Jolla, CA

"In her latest book, Kathryn Simpson has brought to us a wonderful, understandable approach to thyroid dysfunction. As a neurologist and sleep disorders specialist, I am impressed how little the medical community at large investigates this common set of disorders and even more impressed with how passive therapy usually is. With this book as a guide, anyone can easily understand thyroid-related symptoms, be empowered to undergo appropriate testing, and intelligently evaluate the response to replacement therapy."

—Victor Rosenfeld, MD, neurology department head at the Sansum Clinic in Santa Barbara, CA

THE WOMEN'S GUIDE TO
Thyroid Health

Comprehensive Solutions for All Your Thyroid Symptoms

KATHRYN R. SIMPSON, MS

New Harbinger Publications, Inc.

Publisher's Note

A Word of Caution

Distributed in Canada by Raincoast Books

Copyright © 2009 by Kathryn R. Simpson, MS
New Harbinger Publications, Inc.
5674 Shattuck Avenue
Oakland, CA 94609
www.newharbinger.com

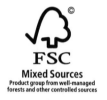

FSC
Mixed Sources
Product group from well-managed
forests and other controlled sources

Cert no. SW-COC-002283
www.fsc.org
© 1996 Forest Stewardship Council

Cover design by Amy Shoup; Acquired by Melissa Kirk; Edited by Jasmine Star; Text design by Tracy Carlson

Library of Congress Cataloging-in-Publication Data

Simpson, Kathryn R.
  The women's guide to thyroid health / Kathryn R. Simpson.
    p. cm.
  Includes bibliographical references.
  ISBN-13: 978-1-57224-577-8 (pbk. : alk. paper)
  ISBN-10: 1-57224-577-8 (pbk. : alk. paper)
  1. Hypothyroidism--Popular works. 2. Women--Diseases--Popular works. 3. Thyroid gland--Popular works. I. Title.
  RC657.S565 2008
  616.4'44--dc22

                              2008052209

11   10   09
10   9   8   7   6   5   4   3   2   1   First printing

Dedicated to all the women who are searching for answers to their thyroid problems. Take heart—there is a solution!

Contents

Foreword

Thyroid hormones are crucial to every single function in your body. You can't survive without them. But as we age, particularly in our current world, we rarely have optimum levels of these and many other important hormones. This means we don't have optimum health and often end up with conditions like arthritis, heart disease, flagging sex drive, gray hair, wrinkles, and ever-increasing weight gain—all signs that may be caused by low thyroid function.

In this book, Kathy Simpson provides a huge amount of information and also illuminates several fundamental truths that may change the way you view your situation. First, she makes clear the overall importance of thyroid hormones for a woman's happiness, health, and even beauty. Second, she focuses on information that's often neglected in the medical world, specifically that thyroid hormones don't work alone. They only work well if appropriate dietary and lifestyle changes are made, if necessary hormone replacement therapy is implemented to correct hormonal and nutritional deficiencies, and if environmental factors support hormone health. For example, your body may not respond well to thyroid therapy if your diet is lacking in important amino acids, if levels of other important hormones are imbalanced, or if you're exposed to toxic chemicals (including mercury amalgam fillings). Factors such as these can compromise your recovery despite adequate thyroid medication.

The Women's Guide to Thyroid Health is definitely a complete guide. It contains all of the important information you'll need to optimize your thyroid function, written in clear, comprehensible language. Because of its incredible thoroughness, it's better not to read it in a hurry. There is too much useful information contained in the book to try to absorb it in one sitting. Take your time and read it bit by bit in order to integrate its valuable information and apply it to your daily living.

—Thierry Hertoghe, MD
President of the International Hormone Society
Author of *The Hormone Handbook, The Patient Hormone Handbook,* and
The Hormone Solution

Acknowledgments

Thanks to the Hertoghe family—doctors Eugene, Luc, Jacques, Therese, and Thierry—who have shaped the way the world thinks about hormones for over a hundred years. To Hiram French, Jo Ann Roland, Debbie Merino, Jasmine Star, Melissa Kirk and the whole New Harbinger bunch, and William Van Valin, MD, for all their help and support. To all the women and doctors who generously shared their stories and experiences. And especially to my family—Bob, Tyler, Kyle, and Myles—who've had to hear more about thyroid function than anyone should have to.

Introduction

Doctors have traditionally been in complete charge of our health, and even our bodies. But this is starting to change as more and more women realize that they can no longer sit passively by and turn their health over to anyone else—even the best-trained doctor. While doctors certainly play a key role in health care, successful patients realize that doctors' orders alone won't make them well—that the relationship with our medical team is a two-way street and that health is primarily the responsibility of the individual. And now, with in-depth medical research readily available on the Internet on even the rarest of medical conditions, you can be fully informed and take charge of your situation to ensure you're getting the best care possible.

As confident as I may sound now, I have to be honest: The need to manage my own health care wasn't always obvious to me. I learned it the hard way after I was diagnosed with multiple sclerosis (MS) eight years ago. It was a long process for me to get to the bottom of what was going on: that low thyroid, adrenal, and ovarian function were at the root of all my symptoms of MS. My path was fraught with many dead ends and false starts as I worked with various doctors to try to figure out what was causing my health problems.

My problems started innocently enough when I was thirty-nine, with numbness in my hands. By forty-three I had also started to experience fatigue, bladder problems, irregular menstrual cycles, hair loss, chronic back pain, and brain fog. I went to my doctor, who listened as I recounted all my symptoms and then said he needed to run some tests for the fatigue but that I would need to see specialists for everything else. He referred me to a neurologist for my numbness, a dermatologist for my hair loss, a urologist for my bladder problems, an orthopedist for my back pain, and an ob-gyn for my menstrual problems. He called me several days later and told me that all my tests results looked normal, and he recommended that I follow up as soon as possible with the specialists.

So I made the appointments, but I was completely discouraged by the outcome: The neurologist said, "It's carpal tunnel syndrome. You need surgery on your hands." The urologist said, "Bladder problems are common after having two children. Surgery should correct it." The orthopedist did an X-ray and said I had degenerative arthritis in my spine, for which there was no treatment. The ob-gyn prescribed birth control pills to try to regulate my cycle and mentioned that, ultimately, a hysterectomy might be required. By then, I was so discouraged at the prospect of all that surgery and continued pain that I didn't even bother with the dermatologist.

Hesitant to undergo invasive surgical procedures, I decided to start with the birth control pills. Unfortunately, they only made me feel worse. After two months I stopped taking them, and I was back to square one. Over the next two years I went from bad to worse, with the numbness that had plagued my hands for years now spreading to the right side of my face. So I went back to the neurologist, who did several more tests and said bluntly, "I think you have multiple sclerosis," and scheduled an MRI and a spinal tap to confirm the diagnosis. Unfortunately, the spinal tap site leaked afterward for almost a week. This insult to my central nervous system launched a whole new set of symptoms, and even more unfortunate, both tests were positive for MS.

By now I had lost virtually all eyesight in my right eye and the left was starting to get blurry, forcing me to get reading glasses in order to use a computer or read. I had such bad back and leg pain that I was unable to walk more than thirty yards without having to crouch down to stretch out the muscles in my lower back. It was almost impossible for me to bend down to pick anything up. My cognitive confusion was such that most of the time I couldn't make sense out of basic math, and balancing my checkbook became a nightmare. I was often so tired that I stopped scheduling activities in the afternoons, as I spent most of them lying down. I had the bladder function of an eighty-year-old, and to top things off I had lost at least half of my hair, my face and lips were pale and drawn, my skin was so dry it was scaly and cracking, and my fingernails were breaking off and getting split and ridged.

The days are pretty much gone when doctors actually look at a patient's body and use physical symptoms to figure out what's going on. So even though I tried many times to interest various doctors in these puzzling changes (which I now know were clearly indicative of low thyroid function) no one ever made the connection because my thyroid function tests were in the "normal" range. This is when I realized that specialists weren't going to fix me, and that I needed to try something different. (As you'll read in chapter 6, it's essential to find a doctor with training and experience in endocrine disorders, or you may end up misdiagnosed, as I was. You may notice that most of the people in the case histories in this book had well-informed doctors. This is because their stories are based on the experiences of patients at a clinic specializing in hormone health.)

Strangely enough, when I finally accepted the fact that doctors weren't going to save me, it gave me a renewed sense of purpose. I had worked in the biotech industry for years and had run large development projects and seen scientific breakthroughs firsthand. Why couldn't I do this myself? But if I was going to be successful, I needed to get organized, particularly given my variable brain function. I sat down and made a complete list of all the symptoms I was experiencing and started to research them systematically. And a strange thing happened: I started to see a common theme emerge from the many disparate symptoms that none of the doctors had thought were related (and certainly not related to my MS). The unifying element was that they were all symptoms of hormone deficiency. From the most obvious—irregular menstrual cycles—to the numbness in my hands and pain in my back, medical research showed they all had hormonal involvement.

I spent the next few months learning everything I could about hormones and finding out that the symptoms of hormone deficiencies and MS are very similar, although the symptoms are obviously much more drastic in MS. I became convinced that correcting deficient hormone levels was a potential solution for my worsening symptoms. I returned to my doctor and went through all of my research with him, including what I had found out about the hormonal nature of my symptoms, and he agreed to test my hormone levels. Sure enough, my estrogen and progesterone levels were extremely low. Strangely, given that so many of my symptoms were indicative of low thyroid function, my thyroid tests were all in the normal ranges. But at least my doctor agreed to write me a prescription for estrogen and progesterone. Within a matter of weeks some of my symptoms started to resolve, and that's when I realized I was on the right track.

This was a start, but many symptoms still remained. Looking back, with the benefit of all I've learned, I can now see that I suffered from thyroid dysfunction for decades. My symptoms were fairly minor until after I had my last child at age forty-one, and then they got much more severe: bladder problems, infertility, chronic fatigue, numbness in my hands and face, constipation, puffy skin, frequent colds, sinusitis, hair loss, brain fog, and cold, dry hands and feet. I had no idea what was causing these symptoms, and I certainly had no clue that it could be an inherited genetic problem. I didn't even stumble onto the thyroid connection until after I was diagnosed with MS.

In discussing my health situation with my family, I told my mother that based on my symptoms, I thought I might have thyroid problems. I was stunned when she told me she had been on thyroid medication since her midforties, and so had her mother and sister. After discovering my inherited predisposition for thyroid disorder, I started to research the connection between thyroid function and MS in earnest. This led me to uncover a lot of research showing the importance of good thyroid function for nerve health. I found one study after another that showed thyroid function to be directly related to nerve health and repair. This is why it's so important for you to complete a family history as part of your analysis of your situation. If I'd known about this genetic link, I would have looked more closely at the thyroid connection earlier, which could have stopped my downward spiral much sooner.

When I finally realized that my symptoms indicated potential low thyroid function, I had my thyroid hormone levels tested. Because my tests were all in the "normal" range, my doctor was hesitant to prescribe thyroid hormones. But my family history gave me the impetus and confidence I needed to continue hounding him for a trial course of thyroid hormone therapy. He finally agreed, based on the fact that the entire maternal line of my family had compromised thyroid function. As it turned out, thyroid dysfunction (central hypothyroidism) was a huge part of my neurological problems, and my symptoms resolved when I started thyroid hormone therapy.

Today, as I write this at age fifty-four, I supplement thyroid, estrogen, progesterone, testosterone, and cortisol, and I have boundless amounts of energy, a sharp mind, a full head of hair, and excellent vision in both eyes—I don't even need reading glasses anymore. My only remaining symptom is a slight residual numbness in my right hand, which I believe also could have been resolved if I'd supplemented my deficient hormones sooner. So, is it MS (or, as I like to call it, "multiple symptoms"), or is it multiple hormone deficiencies? Does it matter what it's called? The bottom line is that often, especially in women, the symptoms of both of these conditions (and many others, such as fibromyalgia and lupus) are suspiciously similar, and there's no reason to suffer either the symptoms of hormonal imbalance or the diseases it can lead to. For me, the answer to restoring my health was taking charge of it myself. By embracing the following advice, you can start to do the same thing.

Be confident. Be assured that you *can* successfully manage your own health and get to the bottom of your disturbing symptoms and resolve them. You're not at the mercy of your doctors or the health care system. You know your body better than anyone else, so when it comes to your health you can't afford to sit passively by.

Be educated. Educate yourself about your physical signs and symptoms before they get significant enough to create serious health problems. The best place to start is by doing the symptom questionnaires in the following chapters. For further information, you can go to an Internet search engine like Google, enter your symptom, and click on "search." You will likely get hundreds if not thousands of pages of information. There's a lot of misleading information out there in addition to the helpful resources, so focus on reputable sources. Take a methodical and organized approach to your research, and to compiling this information so you can share it with your doctor.

Be assertive. To take full responsibility for your health, you may need to be more assertive than you usually are with your health care providers. This may require a departure from the nice, easy-to-manage, suffer-in-silence person you may have been at your doctor's office in the past. An approach you may find useful is the simple "broken record" technique: Repeat yourself over and over until you're taken seriously. Describe your feelings and state your requests using "I" statements, showing your doctor that you take responsibility for yourself; for example, "I would like my thyroid hormone levels tested." Be firm and sure of yourself, remain pleasant, and don't get emotional.

Be positive. Focus on positive goals, such as how empowering it is to take charge of your own health and how great you'll feel when you get rid of your distressing symptoms. Once you learn about your body and start taking charge of your own health, you and your health care providers will become a valuable team!

CHAPTER 1

Why Your Thyroid Gland Is Important

What happened to that report I was almost finished with? Okay ... how did it wind up in my System Preferences folder? And why am I standing in front of this filing cabinet? It's finally lunchtime but where did I put my car keys? Uh-oh, I see "11:30—Lauren" written in my Day-Timer. What does it mean ... and who is Lauren? The dozen or so Post-it notes stuck to my computer screen don't give me a clue. I better leave a message on my voice mail in case she calls to find out where I am. How the heck do I leave a message on voice mail, anyway? Oh, look, my keys are in my bottom drawer ... Now how did they get there?

If this sounds familiar, you could be suffering from brain fog, one of the most common symptoms of *hypothyroidism* ("hypo" means low, so "hypothyroidism" means low thyroid function). Brain fog is a state of confusion that can feel like a cloud shrouding your brain, a sense that you just can't quite think straight or concentrate. You may stare at the paper in front of you or at the task at hand as your thoughts swirl around in your head refusing to focus or make sense, causing you to become forgetful, detached, and often discouraged and depressed. Good thyroid function is critical to concentration and memory. Because low levels of thyroid hormones causes your metabolism to slow down, any deficiency impacts your entire body, including your brain, where it can lead to problems like memory loss and inability to process data.

YOUR THYROID: SMALL GLAND, BIG DEAL

Your thyroid is a miraculous gland. Located at the base of the front of your neck, it produces the hormones that are responsible not just for a sharp mind, but also for the svelte figure and cheerful outlook of our youth. Do you look around and see yourself or friends, family, and strangers your age getting bigger, balder, and more irritable? As we age, many people, especially women, develop low thyroid function, which is reflected in weight gain, hair loss, constipation, dry skin, high cholesterol, fatigue, allergies, breathing problems, impaired vision and hearing, sleeping disorders, dizziness, numbness, loss of libido, aches and pains, more frequent infections, and increasing incidence of mental and emotional problems such as depression, rage, anxiety, irritability, and even schizophrenia and bipolar disorder (De Groot, Hennemann, and Larsen 1984). Let's face it, any of these symptoms would be enough to make us depressed and irritable. Sadly, even though no other hormone affects such a wide range of tissues and cells, our thyroid gets little attention until it seriously malfunctions and causes problems. And even then, most doctors overlook it in their search for clues about what is causing our symptoms.

When our levels of sex hormone start dropping, generally somewhere after age thirty-five, we can start to feel pretty wretched. The telltale signs of incipient aging start to appear: dry and thinning hair, weight gain, loosening skin and wrinkles, irritability...you name it. However, as bad as these symptoms may get, we can still live relatively normal lives even if we slow down and get various strange aches and pains. This is what loss of hormones such as estrogen, progesterone, testosterone, and growth hormone—hormones that are at high levels in our youth—can do to us. But if our thyroid goes, things can really fall apart. Studies done as early as the 1800s showed that when animals' thyroids were removed, they often died within a few days. In the name of science, ovaries, testicles, and various other endocrine glands have been removed from animals over the years, and the animals were able to carry on fairly well. But when French medical researcher Raynard got around to taking out a dog's thyroid gland in 1835 and it promptly died, the medical world finally realized the significance of this tiny gland (Barker, Hoskins, and Mosenthal 1922). When surgeon and anatomist Astley Cooper removed the thyroids of several young pups in 1836, they fared somewhat better than their older counterparts, but he noted they suffered from "stupidity and malaise" (Vincent 1912, 287). Who among us with low thyroid function can't relate to this?

⤺ Cindy's Story

At forty-one, Cindy felt she was starting to lose her mind. The first time something strange occurred was in front of a group of doctors as she was demonstrating a new ultrasound machine for her firm. She had done it a hundred times and usually didn't even have to concentrate on her presentation; she just went through it by rote. But that morning after introducing herself and making a few opening remarks, she just stood there staring blankly. She said it was like a switch had turned off in her mind. Fortunately, she recalled a technique she had been taught in case she froze in a presentation: asking the group if there were any questions. Luckily, the doctors jumped right in and started talking, allowing her to get back on track.

Unfortunately, these incidents of brain fog started to become more and more frequent. Although she never went completely blank again, she had to develop backup systems of Post-it notes and cue cards as she became increasingly forgetful. After she spent more than an hour trying to find her rental car in a parking lot because she couldn't remember its color or make, she began to think that she would have to ask to be transferred into a job that didn't require so much travel and stress. She knew that some of her coworkers had started to notice the change in her and was worried that her boss would be the next to notice.

At the same time as her memory problems were getting worse, she also noticed that she was having a hard time sleeping and was becoming more and more irritable. She just assumed that the irritability was due to the combination of insomnia and the stress her memory problems created. But she didn't realize how bad it had gotten until her husband sat her down and told her that he was concerned about her because her behavior was changing noticeably. She immediately thought the worst. What could be causing such a radical change in her mental function and personality? Could it be a brain tumor?

Fortunately, this thought scared Cindy into immediately making an appointment with her doctor. The history her doctor took pointed out several other changes in Cindy's health that she hadn't focused on, such as chronic constipation and insidious weight gain, which now totaled twenty-five extra pounds. Plus, no matter what the weather, she was always cold. Her doctor connected the dots and told her he was concerned about her thyroid function and sent her for lab tests. When Cindy returned a week later to go over the lab results, her doctor told her that the tests had confirmed his suspicions: Her thyroid function was significantly low. She started on thyroid hormone replacement and noticed a huge difference within the first few weeks. Her thinking and memory were dramatically improved, she slept better from the first night, and the anxiety and irritation that had plagued her for over a year simply disappeared.

HYPOTHYROIDISM—A SURPRISINGLY COMMON AILMENT

Cindy's story isn't unusual. The estimates are staggering: 25 percent of all women develop permanent hypothyroidism, with the greatest incidence occurring after age thirty-four (American Association of Clinical Endocrinologists 2007). Not coincidentally, the midthirties are also when perimenopause usually starts. At this time, we stop ovulating regularly and the resulting decrease in ovarian hormones (specifically estrogen and progesterone) greatly affects the thyroid's ability to do its job. Adolescence and pregnancy are also times of tremendous hormonal flux and likewise are times when thyroid dysfunction is more likely. There is a close relationship between our ovarian function and our thyroid function. Unfortunately, because the symptoms of hypothyroidism are so similar to those of perimenopause and menopause, hypothyroidism is easily missed.

It would be difficult to state the importance of diagnosing hypothyroidism any more articulately than physician Charles Sajous did almost a hundred years ago. He said that hypothyroidism "keeps the patient in a state of perpetual torment [and leaves them] prey to acute suffering from so-called rheumatism, neuralgia, tic douloureaux, sciatica, etc." He went on to say that when these symptoms of thyroid dysfunction aren't diagnosed correctly, "the sufferer finally abandons treatment—at least that offered by medical men" (Sajous 1914, 176-177). How many of us have encountered this? We go hopefully from one doctor to another with our list of symptoms, which may include back pain, joint pain, sciatica, fatigue, headaches, depression, brain fog, and so much more, and then we finally give up because nothing we are given—generally pain pills, antidepressants, or birth control pills—makes much of a difference.

Why is it that almost a century after Sajous's insightful comments we're still in the same place or, let's face it, even worse off than we were back then? At least when there weren't a multitude of pharmaceutical treatments available for each symptom, doctors had to try to get to the root of what was causing the problem and fix it in order to help their patients. Compare that to modern "solutions," where you end up with multiple prescriptions for constipation, depression, cognition problems, fatigue, and weight gain. Many of us are on several different powerful prescription drugs before we are even fifty years old. And let's not forget our ever-expanding store of lotions and creams for dry skin and hair, ever more powerful reading glasses, and mechanical aids such as splints for conditions like carpal tunnel syndrome.

Although we are hearing more about the thyroid in the media recently (particularly since Oprah announced she has hypothyroidism), thyroid disease is not a new phenomenon. Worldwide estimates of the incidence of thyroid dysfunction have been high since the beginning of the twentieth century. In 1976, thyroid expert and researcher Dr. Broda Barnes estimated that 40 percent of people had hypothyroidism (Barnes and Galton 1976), and more recently, Belgian endocrinologist Dr. Jacques Hertoghe suggested the rate could be as high as 80 percent (Durrant-Peatfield 2002). There are many reasons for this prevalence of hypothyroidism: genetic inheritance, diet, our increasingly toxic environment, exposure to certain viruses, iodine deficiency, direct physical trauma to the thyroid, indirect trauma (such as whiplash), autoimmune diseases, thyroid antibodies, and even medical advancements that have allowed more people with hypothyroidism to survive infancy.

This concept of decreased natural selection was studied extensively by Broda Barnes in the 1960s and 1970s. With the introduction of antibiotics in 1944, deaths from infectious diseases were drastically reduced. Prior to the age of antibiotic drugs, the majority of children didn't survive to adulthood. Barnes speculated that 99 percent of children with frequent infections had hypothyroidism, and that once these children were able to survive childhood and reproduce, they ended up spreading hypothyroidism widely in the gene pool, hence the dramatic increase in incidence of hypothyroidism (Barnes and Galton 1976).

Something similar happened with tuberculosis, after drugs that cured it were developed around the same time. In one group of people Barnes studied, there was a large decrease in deaths from infection and tuberculosis between 1930 and 1970, but at the same time there was an enormous increase in deaths from heart attacks, emphysema, prostate cancer, childhood cancers, and lung cancer. Barnes said that the hypothyroid children who survived early life-threatening infections went on to get these and other opportunistic diseases due to their low thyroid function, and hence low immune function (Barnes and Galton 1976).

Should we all panic? Absolutely not! I, my husband, and all three of my children have thyroid problems and have managed to overcome them. There's an easy solution to thyroid problems: Get your thyroid hormone levels tested, and have your children tested if they exhibit any signs of thyroid disease (see chapter 10 for the Children's Thyroid Symptom Evaluation). With your doctor, review your symptoms and test results carefully, then simply take supplemental thyroid hormones if your levels are low. It's one of the easiest hormone deficiencies to correct.

Still, it's frightening that this common and easily treated disease, which can affect almost every aspect of your health, is frequently misunderstood, misdiagnosed, and overlooked. If you're one of the millions of women who intuitively suspect that something is wrong with your thyroid function, now is the time to do something about it. You may already have asked your doctor several times if your thyroid could be at the root of your health problems. Stop wondering. Take charge of your health and find out for sure if your thyroid is the culprit. Few doctors (other than endocrinologists, who specialize in hormones) receive medical training in diagnosing and treating thyroid problems. The unfortunate result is that when you ask your general practitioner or ob-gyn (or whatever doctor you count on for medical advice) about your thyroid health, you're likely to be brushed off with statements such as "Women always think their thyroid is responsible for their weight gain, but this is just an excuse; you just need to change your diet and start exercising" or "Fatigue has nothing to do with your thyroid; you're working too hard" or "You have young children; it's to be expected that you're tired." Meanwhile, the look in their eyes sadly conveys that they suspect you're a hopeless hypochondriac. Some doctors are willing to test thyroid function, but even these may stop short of doing all the tests necessary to give a full picture of how your thyroid is functioning. Plus, many doctors may not understand how to interpret these test results. But this is exactly what's needed if you're to get to the bottom of what's going on once and for all.

UNDERSTANDING YOUR THYROID

In order to understand how your thyroid may be affecting your health, you must first understand how it works. Thyroid hormones are responsible for powering all metabolic processes in our bodies:

- They help maintain constant temperature, which is why the hands and feet are always cold when the thyroid starts to slow down.

- They enable synthesis of protein for normal growth and repair, which is why women with long-standing thyroid deficiency are shorter.

- They help get rid of cellular waste products, which is why low thyroid function leads to accumulation of waste products and results in puffy skin on the face, arms, and thighs.

- They're critical to immune function, which is why we start to get chronic colds and flus when thyroid function is low.

- They stimulate increased blood flow, which is why we get brain fog and cognitive impairment when low thyroid function slows blood flow to the brain.

- They stimulate oxygen consumption in the heart, liver, skeletal muscles, and kidneys. If you've ever spent much time at high altitudes where you didn't get enough oxygen, you know the effect this has: You function poorly and feel weak, sick, and dizzy.

- And finally, they regulate energy production, which is why we get more and more tired when the thyroid isn't working properly.

Your thyroid gland is regulated by your pituitary and hypothalamus, small endocrine glands in your brain. The hypothalamus produces thyrotropin-releasing hormone (TRH), which stimulates the pituitary to release thyroid-stimulating hormone (TSH), which in turn stimulates your thyroid gland to produce four hormones in response to your body's needs: T1 (monoiodotyrosine), T2 (diiodotyrosine), T3 (triiodothyronine), and T4 (thyroxine).

Thyroid stimulation pathway

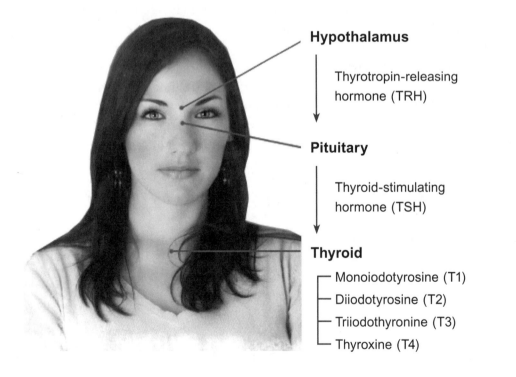

Hypothalamus

Thyrotropin-releasing hormone (TRH)

Pituitary

Thyroid-stimulating hormone (TSH)

Thyroid
- Monoiodotyrosine (T1)
- Diiodotyrosine (T2)
- Triiodothyronine (T3)
- Thyroxine (T4)

Of the four thyroid hormones, blood levels of T4 are the highest—approximately four times higher than levels of T3. However, T3 is far more potent and biologically active than the others. The body makes a lot of T4 and converts it to T3 as needed. T2 hasn't been well understood until fairly recently, when research clarified that it stimulates enzymes critical to producing T3. T2 has also been shown to increase metabolism in the liver, heart, muscle tissue, and fat tissue. As it's been found to break down fat without breaking down muscle tissue, T2 has recently found its way into weight-loss supplements. It's also been proven that T2 stimulates oxygen uptake and increases overall metabolic rate (Lanni et al. 2005). Lastly, T1 is still somewhat of a mystery, but it is thought to control the electrical input and charge of the brain in some way (Lanni et al. 1998; Goglia and DeLange 2003).

Your thyroid can malfunction in two basic ways: It can become underactive, resulting in hypothyroidism. Or, more rarely, it can become overactive, resulting in *hyperthyroidism* ("hyper" means excessive, so "hyperthyroidism" means excessive thyroid function). When T3 and T4 levels drop too low, the pituitary gland responds by making more thyroid-stimulating hormone, which does exactly what its name suggests: It stimulates your thyroid to produce more T3 and T4. Increasing TSH levels mean that your thyroid hormone levels are dropping. The picture gets even more complex when you realize that your thyroid gland also works in close concert with all of the other parts of your endocrine system (described in the next chapter), so this system must also be functioning adequately in order for your thyroid to do its job.

Symptoms and Signs of Hypothyroidism

Anxiety	Deafness or hearing	Hemorrhoids
Asthma	problems	High blood pressure
Attention-deficit/	Decreased sex drive	Hoarse voice
hyperactivity disorder	Depression	Infertility
Back or leg pain	Dry, coarse skin	Insomnia and sleep
Bladder irritation	Early menopause	problems
Bluish skin, nail beds, lips,	Easy bruising	Intolerance of cold or heat
or mucous membranes	Eczema or psoriasis	Lack of sweating
Bowel problems	Elevated cholesterol	Listless, dull eyes
Brain fog and memory	Enlarged abdomen	Liver pain or swelling
problems	Excessive fatigue	Looking older than your age
Breathlessness	Fibrocystic breast disease	Loss of body hair
Brittle, thin, ridged	Fibromyalgia	Low basal body temperature
fingernails	Flatulence	Low blood pressure
Carpal tunnel syndrome	Food cravings	Muscle weakness
Cervical dysplasia	Hair loss	Pain in the hands and feet
Chronic colds and illness	Halitosis	Painful or irregular periods
Chronic constipation	Headaches	Pale lips
Cold hands and feet	Heart enlargement	Pale or yellow skin
	Heart palpitations	PMS

Puffy face and eyelids	Strange thoughts and	Tinnitus
Recurrent upper	psychological problems	Urinary urgency and
respiratory and urinary	Swollen legs and feet	frequency
tract infections	Thickening of the neck or	Vision problems
Restless legs syndrome	goiter	Voice changes
Scalloped, thick, or wasting	Thinning, dry, coarse,	Weak, slow, or soft pulse
tongue	brittle hair	Weight gain
Slow speech	Thinning eyebrows, espe-	Yeast infections
Slowed Achilles reflex	cially at the outer ends	Yellowish skin or whites
Sluggish movement	Tingling in the hands and	of the eyes
Stiffness and pain	feet	

Common Symptoms and Signs of Hyperthyroidism

Breathlessness	Increased bowel movements	Red, irritated eyes
Fatigue or feeling wired but	Insomnia	Staring gaze
tired	Irritability	Thickening of the skin over
Feeling overheated much of	Light or absent menstrual	the lower legs
the time	periods	Trembling hands
Hair loss	Muscle weakness	Warm, moist skin
Heart palpitations or fast	Nervousness	Weight loss
heart rate	Protruding eyes	

WHAT'S NEXT?

Having a basic understanding of how your thyroid functions is vital in order to successfully work with your doctor to figure out if any physical symptoms you're having could be caused by thyroid dysfunction. It's also an important basis for grasping the complexities of thyroid testing and treatment if this becomes necessary.

Now that you understand how your thyroid gland functions, you need to understand it in the context of the rest of your endocrine system. For your thyroid gland to do its job, the other glands must do theirs. Problems with any of the other endocrine glands will affect your thyroid function. The next chapter gives you an overview of the endocrine system, which is a sophisticated and elegant system with many built-in checks and balances.

KEY POINTS

 Symptoms of hypothyroidism are many and varied. They include weight gain, hair loss, constipation, dry skin, high cholesterol, fatigue, allergies, breathing problems, impaired vision and hearing, sleeping disorders, dizziness, numbness, loss of libido, aches and pains, more frequent infections, and increasing incidence of mental and emotional problems such as depression, rage, anxiety, irritability, and even schizophrenia and bipolar disorder.

Experts have suggested many different estimates of rates of hypothyroidism, some as high as 40 to 80 percent of the population. Causes of hypothyroidism include genetic inheritance, diet, our increasingly toxic environment, exposure to certain viruses, iodine deficiency, direct physical trauma to the thyroid, indirect trauma (such as whiplash), autoimmune diseases, thyroid antibodies, and even medical advancements that have allowed more people with hypothyroidism to survive infancy.

The introduction of antibiotics and other drugs in the earlier part of the twentieth century prevented deaths from infectious diseases that often resulted from low thyroid function. This has undoubtedly resulted in hypothyroidism becoming more widespread in the gene pool, causing an increase in incidence of hypothyroidism.

Your thyroid gland is regulated by your pituitary and hypothalamus. Problems with either of these glands, as well as the thyroid gland itself, can result in thyroid dysfunction.

CHAPTER 2

The Endocrine System and How It Affects Your Thyroid

There are nine major glands in the endocrine system: the pineal gland, hypothalamus, pituitary, thyroid, parathyroid glands, thymus, adrenals, pancreas, and reproductive glands (ovaries and testes). Together, they make over one hundred hormones. Through this handful of glands and the hormones they produce, the endocrine system regulates, coordinates, and controls an extraordinary number of body functions.

The word "hormone" comes from the Greek word *hormon*, which means to stir up, excite, or spur on, and that's exactly what they do: They cause other things to happen. Countless numbers of these amazing hormones are always busily directing and regulating such things as your mood, when you feel hungry or full, how you sleep, your body temperature, how you digest and utilize the food you eat, your weight, how you handle stress, and when you start puberty, perimenopause, and menopause and how long these processes take. Many of us think our genes determine these things, but it really depends on our hormones. The amounts of the different hormones we produce are definitely genetically programmed, but many other factors also affect hormonal activity, including diet, exercise, sleep, exposure to environmental toxins, and substance use or abuse.

In general, the endocrine system is in charge of processes in your body that happen slowly, such as cell growth. Activities that occur more quickly, like movement, are controlled by your nervous system. Your nervous system uses electricity to orchestrate all sorts of activities in your body, and your endocrine system does even more through the miracle of hormones, which use your bloodstream to communicate information. Each hormone is designed to affect only certain cells called *target cells*. These target cells have receptors for specific hormones. When the hormones reach their target cells via your blood, they lock onto the cell's receptors and transmit instructions, which cause amazing things to occur: breasts grow, hips widen, hair grows lush and shiny, and skin glows.

An interesting experiment done in the early days of endocrinology first showed us how hormones operate. In 1849, physiologist Arnold Berthold castrated four young male chickens. Two of the castrated chickens were left effectively chicken eunuchs, but he transplanted the testes back into the other two at a site distant from their normal location. The two eunuch chickens never developed male characteristics, but the chickens that received transplanted testes matured into normal adult male roosters (Soma 2006). This experiment demonstrated that hormones can access the bloodstream from any site and still function correctly. In fact, fragments of thyroid tissue about the size of a grain of wheat were commonly grafted to different parts of the body as a treatment for hypothyroidism. These grafts were able to carry on thyroid functions quite well for a short period of time, but then the tissue was absorbed by the body and the procedure had to be repeated (Sajous 1922; Sajous and Sajous 1930).

PARTS OF THE ENDOCRINE SYSTEM

Too much or too little of any hormone can be harmful to your body, and the elements of your endocrine system work together to ensure you have the right levels of each. For example, if your thyroid has made the right amount of thyroid hormones, your pituitary gland senses this and adjusts the amount of thyroid-stimulating hormone it releases; this type of process is called a *negative feedback system*.

Overall, your endocrine system is governed by this sophisticated system of checks and balances. For your thyroid to do its job, your hypothalamus, located in the center of the brain, must tell your pituitary, located just below it, what to do. The pituitary, in turn, tells your other endocrine glands what to do. Problems with any of these glands will affect your thyroid.

Because I spent many years in the corporate world, I find it helpful to think of the endocrine system in terms of a company's structure. The hypothalamus is the body's chief executive officer; it has overall management responsibility and interfaces with the outside world, detecting things such as ambient temperature and light. The pituitary is the chief operating officer; it runs internal operations and coordinates interactions between all of the different functional areas. The rest of the glands are the executive staff and carry out the chief operating officer's directions. Let's take a closer look at these nine endocrine glands, starting at the top.

The Pineal Gland

Physically, the pineal gland is at the top of your endocrine system. In many primitive animals, such as some reptiles, the pineal gland is so close to the skin on the top of the head that it actually responds to outside light. It was once considered a vestigial organ, like the appendix, which also isn't a useless, vestigial organ, but rather an important part of the immune system. One theory was that the pineal gland had been a third eye; in any case, it was believed to no longer be functional or necessary.

But in the 1960s, research found that the pineal gland has many critical functions, including producing melatonin, an extremely important hormone. In humans, the pineal gland isn't near enough to the surface of the body to actually detect light, so it uses the eyes to receive input. The amount of melatonin you produce is based on the amount of light that hits your eyes. As light increases, it causes your pineal gland to reduce the amount of melatonin it makes, so melatonin levels are low during the day and increase to a peak when it's dark. During winter, when the nights are longer, you make more melatonin. This response to light is translated into your body's *circadian rhythm*, daily cycles of physiological and biochemical activity sometimes also called your biological clock (Stokkan and Reiter 1994).

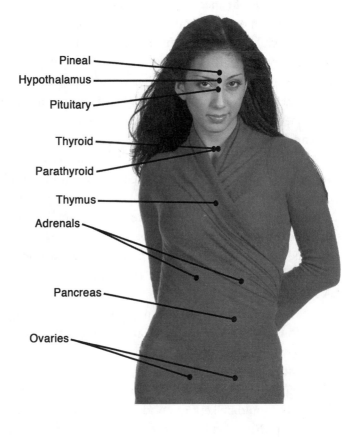

The primary endocrine glands

Pineal
Hypothalamus
Pituitary
Thyroid
Parathyroid
Thymus
Adrenals
Pancreas
Ovaries

This is all well and good, but why do we care about melatonin and why in the world do we need to understand when it's produced? It's important because melatonin has many crucial functions: It helps regulate sleep, it acts as a potent antioxidant, it controls the spread of melanin (the pigment that gives color to skin and hair), and it has several regulatory effects on other hormones. It's well-known that the sun's light directly influences the menstrual cycle. In fact, the survival of many species of animals, such as cows and horses, depends on restricting birth to the spring to increase chances of survival for offspring. The pineal gland appears to be able to judge the season from the length and/or intensity of sunlight.

Melatonin is named for melanin as well as serotonin, a neurotransmitter found abundantly in the pineal gland. Melatonin is made from serotonin, for which the pineal gland appears to be the main reservoir. As it gets dark, serotonin is converted to melatonin, and serotonin levels decrease as a result. As daylight approaches, the increasing light decreases melatonin levels, allowing serotonin to increase. This inverse relationship between serotonin and melatonin helps to explain the condition called seasonal affective disorder (SAD). Studies have shown that, during the winter months, people with SAD have consistently higher daytime melatonin levels and lower serotonin levels, causing symptoms of serotonin deficiency, including depression.

Although it's not terribly realistic to think of hopping into bed as soon as it gets dark, as in the days before electricity, compelling research does suggest that using artificial light at night causes melatonin production to be suppressed and may lead to an increased risk of cancer (Blask et al. 2005). Studies of cancer rates in different societies show that the highest rates occur in the societies that use the most artificial light at night (Rajaratnam and Arendt 2001). There are obviously many other possible reasons for this increased cancer rate, but studies of night shift workers also support this theory. Harvard University researchers found that nurses who worked the night shift at least three times a month for fifteen years or more were 35 percent more likely to develop colon cancer than nurses who never worked nights (Schernhammer et al. 2003). Additionally, studies show that blind people, who make melatonin all the time, have a 30 percent lower rate of all types of cancer (Mann 2002).

Scientists at North Carolina State University conducted an interesting study on ovarian cancer and light. Working with turkey hens, they found that shorter nights with only eight hours of darkness caused ovarian cancer tumors to grow larger. However, when they lengthened the nights to sixteen hours, the tumors became smaller and, in some cases, disappeared completely. They found that reexposure to shorter nights caused tumors to grow back to their former size, leading them to conclude that ovarian cancer in turkeys could be completely manipulated by light exposure (Moore and Siopes 2004). Obviously we aren't turkeys, but clinical studies with humans show similar trends (Vijayalaxmi et al. 2002).

Many scientists believe that cancer is caused by damage to DNA from highly penetrating radiation such as X-rays. Melatonin destroys free radicals produced by this radiation, so it's likely that melatonin's antioxidant properties are an important element in cancer protection. In support of this idea, melatonin has also been shown to inhibit the growth of prostate cancer cells (Sainz et al. 2005). Additional research is needed to fully understand the pineal gland's role in cancer, but two facts should be kept in mind: The first is that light causes the pineal gland to stop making melatonin, and the second is that melatonin inhibits cancer. We should all consider this when we sleep with nightlights on or with streetlights right outside our windows. Try to avoid as much artificial light as possible when you sleep to get the most benefit from your melatonin production.

Just like every other gland in your endocrine system, your pineal gland is inextricably linked to your thyroid. Adequate thyroid activity is necessary for the pineal gland to work correctly, and low thyroid function results in a significant reduction in the amount of melatonin produced (Belviranli 2006). Now that you understand how critical melatonin is, it should come as no surprise that low thyroid function has such profound systemic effects.

The Hypothalamus

Coming next, right under your pineal gland, is your hypothalamus, which plays a critical role by serving as the interface between your endocrine system and the outside world. It tells your pituitary to release various hormones that influence functions essential to life, such as breathing, blood pressure, and heart rate. It also affects critical activities like food intake, weight regulation, awareness of pleasure and pain, metabolism of fats and carbohydrates, sugar levels in the blood, fluid intake and balance, thirst, body temperature, and sleep cycle. When something goes wrong with your hypothalamus, it affects your pituitary and can cause problems with any of the glands the pituitary controls, including your thyroid, resulting in numerous and diverse problems ranging from diabetes, insomnia, and temperature fluctuations to sexual problems and emotional extremes such as fear and rage. Despite the magnitude of its role and the many vital functions it influences, it's only about the size of an almond.

The Pituitary Gland

Your pituitary gland, located just beneath the hypothalamus, roughly behind your nose, is even smaller than your hypothalamus. It's about the size of a pea! Even so, it's one of the most important parts of the endocrine system because it produces hormones that control your other endocrine glands. Its ability to make hormones is affected by many things, including emotions and changes in seasons. It receives information such as emotional state, environmental temperature, and light patterns from the hypothalamus and uses this data to regulate the activity of other glands by producing hormones that stimulate production of even more hormones. Here are some examples of hormones the pituitary produces and their effects:

- Adrenocorticotropic hormone (ACTH) stimulates your adrenals to produce gluco-corticoids, primarily cortisol, in response to stress.

- Luteinizing hormone (LH) and follicle-stimulating hormone (FSH) stimulate your ovaries to make estrogen, progesterone, and testosterone.

- Thyroid-stimulating hormone (TSH), of course, stimulates your thyroid to produce thyroid hormones.

- Growth hormone stimulates growth of bone and other body tissues and helps you utilize nutrients and minerals.

- Prolactin stimulates milk production in breastfeeding women and also has a modulatory role in immune function.

- Oxytocin triggers contractions of the uterus in childbirth and also functions as a neurotransmitter. These days, it's gaining recognition as the "love hormone" or "trust hormone" because it appears to exert a positive effect on our ability to bond with others.

- Vasopressin, an antidiuretic hormone, helps control the balance of water in the body.

The Thyroid Gland

A healthy thyroid gland is critical for a healthy endocrine system and for your overall hormone health. It's responsible for regulating all of your metabolic functions, which isn't just about how you digest food or whether you gain weight; it's about all energy production and use in your body—in every tissue and every cell.

Your thyroid makes hormones that increase the activity and even the numbers of *mitochondria*, the energy generators in every cell that power your body by converting what you eat into body heat and energy. Thyroid hormones control the rate at which oxygen gets into your cells to fuel your brain, heart, muscles, and other organs. They also affect the chemistry of your brain, which affects your mental function, moods, and emotions.

When thyroid function is low, the resulting decrease in energy production causes your body to conserve energy and focus its efforts on essential functions, like repair and regeneration, rather than nonessential functions. This results in a myriad of symptoms. If your hair is falling out, your libido is gone, your skin is so dry that no amount of moisturizer helps, or your mind seems to be playing tricks on you, it could be due to low thyroid function.

Even though these symptoms aren't life-threatening, they're still distressing, especially because they're so widespread. The list of symptoms of low thyroid function makes a compelling case for the importance of resolving thyroid problems: weight gain, fatigue, accelerated aging, constipation, joint and muscle pain, depression, anxiety, back or leg pain, bladder problems, increased susceptibility to illness, elevated cholesterol, headaches, sleep problems, and many, many more. And since thyroid function is closely intertwined with the rest of your endocrine system, it affects the production of all the hormones made by other glands as well, including growth hormone, cortisol, estrogen, and progesterone.

∠ *My Story*

Understanding the relationship between the hypothalamus, pituitary, and thyroid glands was critical in understanding and repairing my own health. When I started trying to get to the bottom of my troubling symptoms, I was suspicious that I had thyroid problems because so many of my symptoms were classic symptoms of hypothyroidism. But every time I had the standard thyroid hormone tests done, I was told my thyroid was fine. These tests (generally a TSH test and sometimes a T4 test) are primarily useful in detecting primary hypothyroidism, where something has gone wrong with the thyroid gland itself.

Unfortunately, if something goes awry with your hypothalamus or pituitary gland, your TSH generally remains at normal levels even if you don't have enough thyroid hormones for your body's needs. This is because some malfunction causes your hypothalamus or pituitary to fail to respond to dropping levels of thyroid hormones by increasing production of the regulatory hormones (TSH in the case of the pituitary and TRH in the case of the hypothalamus), which would result in increased activity of the thyroid gland. Even a slight increase or decrease in thyroid hormone levels can alter the activity in your cells and wreak havoc on your body.

When I finally understood the relationship between the glands, I realized that my very low TSH level coupled with low T3 and T4 levels showed that I had a problem with my hypothalamus and/or pituitary function. This is called central hypothyroidism, and unfortunately, most doctors don't know it exists so they never test for it. Luckily, it responds to thyroid supplementation just like primary hypothyroidism does, and once I started taking supplemental thyroid hormones, all my symptoms of low thyroid function resolved.

The Parathyroid Glands

Attached to your thyroid are four tiny, pea-shaped glands called the parathyroid glands. With the help of calcitonin, produced in the thyroid, they regulate the level of calcium and phosphate in your bones and blood. In addition to promoting strong, healthy bones, they ensure optimum heart function, as calcium is needed for the electrical impulses that cause your heart to beat. These little glands don't get much attention, but you'll develop a better appreciation for them when you consider all that can go wrong when the balance of calcium is upset: muscle cramping and spasms, confusion, depression, and tingling or pins-and-needles sensations in the fingers and around the mouth, not to mention osteoporosis.

Good thyroid function is very important in getting the most out of your parathyroids, as deficient thyroid hormones have been shown to blunt the responsiveness of bone to parathyroid hormone—clearly a danger in developing osteoporosis (Castro, Genuth, and Klein 1975).

The Thymus

As with the pineal gland, few recognized the importance of the thymus until fairly recently, but it's now known to be the body's key regulator of immunity. It oversees the development of a particular type of immune system cell: T lymphocytes, or T cells, which help your body identify and destroy invading bacteria, viruses, and abnormal cells, as in cancer. For years the thymus was thought to be a temporary organ that reached its largest size at puberty and then gradually dwindled until it disappeared at adulthood. The truth of the matter is that the thymus shrivels up in response to factors that cause much of the "aging" process, such as stress, disease, radiation, and malnutrition. In fact, the thymus can shrink to half its size in twenty-four hours due to acute physical stress or serious illness or infection.

Research has shown that although normal aging causes the thymus to shrink in size, it must remain active throughout life and continue to produce lymphocytes for us to remain healthy (Kendall 1984). Levels of thymus hormones drop significantly in hypothyroidism, so it appears that low thyroid function hastens the loss of our thymus function (Hrynevych et al. 2002). An interesting study done by researchers in Israel showed that when thymus extract was given to mice that had their thymus glands removed, immune function was restored (Trainin and Linker-Israeli 1976). Similarly, thymus extracts have been used successfully in humans to resolve serious illnesses (Diamond 1985).

When the thymus is removed or destroyed, the immune system, which guards against infection and cancer, becomes compromised. Studies have shown that the survival rate of mice with tumors was significantly increased by treatment with thymus hormone (Klein et al. 1987). Anecdotal evidence suggests the same may be true in humans. The loss of thymus function may be one of the important reasons why cancer incidence increases with age.

The Adrenal Glands

You have two adrenal glands, one on top of each kidney, which are responsible for producing several critical hormones, including cortisol and adrenaline. These hormones are responsible for controlling how your body manages physical and emotional stress. Cortisol is critical to good health and is produced continuously, but it's also considered a stress hormone, as it's produced in higher amounts when you perceive a threat to your well-being or survival. When you're under any kind of stress—either good stress, such as excitement, or bad stress, such as trauma or illness—your adrenals increase their production of cortisol. This sends a burst of energy that helps you survive any difficulties you might encounter, which in the past generally involved life-threatening things, such as fighting or fleeing from hostile tribes or carnivorous beasts. Cortisol elevates your heart rate, breathing rate, and blood pressure, providing more oxygen and nutrients to your body to help you survive the crisis. At the same time, less critical activities like tissue repair, digestion, hormone production, and immune function are slowed, since they aren't critical to the perceived emergency at hand.

Even if the challenge in front of you is less traumatic than a neighboring tribe on the warpath—but is instead just the busybody next door—your body doesn't know the difference. It still goes through the same physiological changes to send you immediate energy. When the increase in cortisol levels is short-lived, there's no harm done. Unfortunately, if you're under stress for a long period of time, your adrenals finally get exhausted by their endless cortisol production and you end up with something called *adrenal fatigue.* As a result, you feel achy and even more tired, feel cold all the time, get sick more often, get allergies you never had before, lose your stamina, and have blood sugar regulation problems that result in food cravings and weight gain.

To compound the demands on your adrenals, cortisol not only manages your body's response to stress, it also regulates the effects and interactions of other hormones. If your adrenals are fatigued, there isn't enough cortisol to do everything that's needed, so the body has to prioritize what gets done and what doesn't, and producing and managing hormones takes a backseat to survival.

Adrenal function becomes increasingly important as you age. As production of estrogen and progesterone by the ovaries slows down, your adrenals become responsible for backup production of these critical hormones. So your adrenal status is one of the deciding factors in what your path through perimenopause and menopause is like. Rebalancing or rebuilding your adrenal function takes a concerted effort. But a quick review of the symptoms caused by adrenal malfunction should convince you it's worth it: extreme fatigue, difficulty exercising, muscle and joint aches, hypoglycemia, alcoholism, anxiety or panic attacks, allergies, asthma, and more frequent or severe infections.

Your adrenals are also inextricably linked to your thyroid, so adrenal fatigue and thyroid deficiency go hand in hand. Damaged or exhausted adrenals are unable to produce enough cortisol, which is necessary for production of thyroid hormones, conversion of T4 to T3, and fund thyroid receptors. Conversely, if your thyroid isn't functioning well, the resulting slowdown metabolism slows your adrenal function as well. Many doctors who treat thyroid disorders that a large percentage of women with low thyroid function also suffer from adrenal fatigue. So if you have symptoms of low thyroid function, you should always have your adrenal function evaluated as well. This connection is so important that chapter 9 is devoted entirely to the adrenals. There you'll find the Adrenal Fatigue Symptom Evaluation, simple home tests for adrenal function, and an overview of necessary lab tests, treatment, and ways to support your adrenal function.

The Pancreas

Your pancreas produces the hormones insulin and glucagon, as well as digestive enzymes. Insulin's primary job is to move glucose, otherwise known as blood sugar, out of the bloodstream and into fat or muscle cells to be stored for later use. What you eat profoundly affects your insulin and blood sugar levels. Refined carbohydrates, such as candy, soft drinks, cookies, cake, pastries, doughnuts, and even fruit juices, as well as breads, pasta, cereals, and other foods made with white flour, are converted into blood sugar much more quickly than complex carbohydrates (whole grains and products made from them, beans, vegetables, and many fruits).

Blood sugar is stored in your muscle cells until they get full. When this happens, these cells refuse to accept any more glucose, so the body stores it in your fat cells to try to get it out of circulation. You make extra insulin to try to manage the additional glucose, which causes your blood sugar to plunge and leads to blood sugar swings, which results in cravings for caffeine, sugar, and more simple carbs. So remember: The more refined carbohydrates you eat, the more insulin you produce, and the more insulin you produce, the fatter you get.

This vicious cycle also leads to problems more serious than just weight gain. You can develop *insulin resistance*, a condition in which the body loses its ability to respond normally to insulin, and that may lead to type 2 diabetes. In insulin resistance, the normal process of insulin production and blood sugar management breaks down. After being assaulted by years of poor diet, insulin receptors become less functional, so the body can't handle glucose as effectively. In response to the resulting continued high glucose levels, the brain signals your pancreas to release ever-greater amounts of insulin in an attempt to lower blood sugar levels. Insulin resistance is made worse by high cortisol levels and causes significant weight gain (particularly around your middle section), as well as compromised immune function and increased risk of heart disease. Estrogen deficiency exacerbates this situation, as this hormone plays an important role in optimizing insulin response in your cells.

Finally, your thyroid plays an important role in managing insulin. Clinical studies have shown that hypothyroidism increases insulin secretion, so treating hypothyroidism may help normalize insulin production and possibly help prevent the development of diabetes (Lenzen, Joost, and Hasselblatt 1976).

The Reproductive Glands

Our ovaries produce eggs and are our main source of sex hormones: estrogen, progesterone, and testosterone. You're born with your entire life supply of eggs. Most of us start out with about two million eggs, but by our mid- to late thirties we have only about 3 percent left because with age, as well as every time we ovulate, our supply shrinks, reducing estrogen and progesterone levels. Most of us know the obvious effects of estrogen, the primary ovarian hormone. It's responsible for our uniquely feminine shape, particularly our breasts and hips, and it prepares us for pregnancy. It keeps us fertile, agile, and smart and is necessary for almost every function in the body and brain. It triggers the growth of cells and neurons to maintain a good memory and sharp mind, great sex drive, plenty of energy, a healthy heart, good bones, and a cheerful, calm outlook on life, as well as ideal weight and clear, smooth skin.

Estrogen is also necessary for your body to use progesterone effectively. In fact, one of its functions is to create progesterone receptors. Although progesterone was once thought to be involved only in pregnancy, we now know that progesterone receptors occur all over the body, indicating that progesterone is a vital hormone for many functions. Areas with progesterone receptors include the reproductive tract, breasts, skin, hair, urinary tract, heart, blood vessels, bones, mucous membranes, pelvic muscles, and brain (Nash, Morrison, and Frankel 2003).

Thyroid hormones have a mutually dependent relationship with estrogen and progesterone, as indicated by the fact that your ovaries have receptors for thyroid hormones, and your thyroid has receptors for estrogen and progesterone. As early as 1900, it was recognized that their functions were interdependent, and in 1922, pioneering endocrinologist Harry Harrower wrote, "Thyroid disorder is so very commonly associated with menstrual functions that the gynecologist should never consider a case of menstrual derangement without also considering the thyroid function" (Harrower 1922, 32).

It's safe to say that this concept has been lost to the modern world of gynecology. I've never met a gynecologist who looks at thyroid function when a woman complains of common menstrual disorders, such as heavy bleeding. This makes sense when you consider that obstetrics and gynecology is a surgical specialty, so these physicians look for surgical solutions to problems. Is it then any surprise that hysterectomies and uterine ablations are the most common solutions for the heavy bleeding commonly experienced at perimenopause? Tragically for women who take this path, research shows that this condition can often be resolved with thyroid supplementation instead. It's certainly worth exploring before opting for surgery.

Hypothyroidism is far more common in perimenopause and menopause when ovarian function starts to slow down and become erratic. One reason is the mutual dependence between the thyroid and the ovaries. Another reason is the effect that an imbalance between estrogen and progesterone can have on your thyroid. We start to produce less and less progesterone as we stop ovulating regularly, usually sometime after age thirty-five. When this occurs, our estrogen levels aren't balanced by adequate progesterone, so we end up with too much estrogen relative to progesterone. This concept is explained in greater depth in later chapters; for now, the short version is that the resulting condition, sometimes called estrogen dominance, results in elevated levels of certain proteins that suppress both the production and the activity of thyroid hormones and the function of thyroid hormone receptors. Estrogen dominance causes the kinds of symptoms you'd expect to see when the body has too much estrogen, the hormone that causes cells to proliferate: heavy, painful periods and weight gain. Balancing estrogen with progesterone is often the key to rebalancing your thyroid and returning it to normal function.

WHAT'S NEXT?

Now that you understand the basics and interactions of your major endocrine glands, it will be easier to figure out what's going on with your thyroid gland. The next chapter provides symptom evaluations for hypothyroidism and hyperthyroidism so you can start to evaluate if you have thyroid dysfunction, and whether your thyroid is overactive or underactive.

KEY POINTS

🦶 Your endocrine system is in charge of making sure you have optimal levels of all hormones, as too much or too little of any hormone can be harmful to your body. The hypothalamus and pituitary manage a sophisticated system of checks and balances to keep all hormones, including thyroid hormones, at optimal levels and in balance.

🦶 Your pineal gland produces melatonin based on the amount of light that hits your eye. As light increases, your pineal gland reduces the amount of melatonin it makes, so melatonin levels are low during the day and increase to a peak at night. Melatonin regulates sleep, acts as a potent antioxidant, controls the spread of melanin, and has important regulatory effects on other hormones.

🦶 Your hypothalamus plays a critical role in your endocrine system. It's the interface between this system and the outside world. It tells your pituitary to release various hormones that influence activities essential to life, such as breathing, blood pressure, and heart rate.

🦶 Your pituitary regulates the activity of the other glands by producing hormones that stimulate production of additional hormones in the other endocrine glands.

🦶 Your thyroid gland is responsible for regulating all metabolic functions in your body.

🦶 Your parathyroid glands regulate the level of calcium and phosphate in your bones and blood with the help of calcitonin, which is produced in your thyroid. They ensure strong, healthy bones and optimum heart function, as calcium is needed for the electrical impulses that cause your heart to beat.

🦶 The thymus is your body's key regulator of immunity.

🦶 Your adrenal glands are responsible for producing several critical hormones, including cortisol and adrenaline. These hormones are responsible for controlling how your body manages physical and emotional stress.

🦶 Your pancreas produces the hormones insulin and glucagon, as well as digestive enzymes. Insulin's primary job is to move glucose out of the bloodstream and into fat or muscle cells to be stored for later use.

🦶 Our ovaries produce eggs and are our main source of sex hormones: estrogen, progesterone, and testosterone.

CHAPTER 3

Assessing Your Thyroid Health

Take this simple quiz to see if you may have hypothyroidism:

You're convinced that winters have become much colder than they used to be, and the summers hotter!

The dryer has shrunk all of your clothes.

The ability to balance your checkbook is a thing of the past.

Your memory has given out. Post-it notes rule your life.

You're sure that everyone is out to get you or is trying to drive you crazy.

Everyone around you seems to have an attitude problem.

You've revised your definition of a great night in bed to eight hours of medication-free sleep.

Your friends have started to roll their eyes whenever you start to say something.

Your husband and children are suddenly agreeing to everything you say; or, alternatively, your husband and children have turned into complete idiots.

You don't care where your husband goes anymore (or with whom), just as long as you don't have to go with him.

You have stopped trying to hold your stomach in, no matter whom you run into.

You've given up every bad habit you used to have and you still don't feel well.

Almost everything hurts, and anything that doesn't hurt doesn't seem to work.

In all seriousness, if you answered yes to even one of these questions, you've experience first-hand how important a healthy thyroid is to a sound mind and body. Though there are many other possible explanations for any of these phenomena, all of them could be explained by thyroid dysfunction. As you've begun to see, the thyroid affects everything from emotional equanimity, which keeps us from flying off the handle at the slightest little thing, to mental functions like being able to concentrate and remember things, to countless physical effects, from energy level to weight to immune function. Evaluating your thyroid function to get to the bottom of potential problems is probably one of the most important things you can do for your body and your health.

WHY IT'S IMPORTANT TO PAY ATTENTION TO YOUR SYMPTOMS

Physical signs and symptoms are the body's way of communicating what's going on with your health. Your body will give you almost all the information you need to understand what's happening, if you observe it carefully. It's when we ignore these indicators that we get into trouble, yet all too often, that's just what we do. Women tend to stoically bear physical challenges. We get used to suffering from menstrual pain and discomfort at an early age, then to the challenges of pregnancy and the considerable pain of childbirth, followed by the physical demands of nursing. And eventually we face what can be the ultimate challenge—menopause. All of these things are just part of being a woman, so we grow up accepting them and learning to accommodate to them.

When we hit a bump in the road—whether it's fatigue, pain, depression, or simply unusually heavy menstrual periods—we tell ourselves that life must go on: the house has to be cleaned, everyone has to eat, the kids have to be ferried here and there, and endless other tasks must be done—not to mention our jobs if we work outside the house. With all of these responsibilities, we don't have the latitude to give in to physical discomfort. In fact, we may not even want to acknowledge physical problems because we honestly don't have the time (and often don't have the financial means) to try to get to the bottom of what's going on.

As you can imagine, this approach usually backfires. Ignoring the signs and symptoms of deteriorating health doesn't make the problem go away as we so optimistically hope. Just the opposite, it often causes our situation to escalate. In the long run, ignoring physical problems can be very costly at many levels. A much easier and more productive path is to look carefully at the symptoms you're experiencing and explore what these important clues may be telling you about your overall health. You can use this valuable information to chart a path back to your happy, healthy former self. Completing the assessments in this chapter is one of the most important things you can do to determine what's going on in your body and what your symptoms say about how your thyroid is functioning. This will give you and your doctor important insights into your thyroid status and help you determine whether you may have a thyroid condition that needs to be treated.

The lists of symptoms at the end of chapter 1 probably gave you a pretty good idea of whether your thyroid gland is underactive or overactive. Some of the signs and symptoms in the evaluations represent risk factors, rather than symptoms per se. In addition, some of these symptoms can be caused by other hormonal imbalances, with or without thyroid involvement. It's important to look at levels of all of your hormones to understand how your endocrine system is functioning. To evaluate your levels of other key hormones, consult my earlier book, *The Perimenopause and Menopause Workbook* (Simpson and Bredesen 2006).

EXERCISE: Hypothyroidism Symptom Evaluation

This test will help you determine whether your thyroid gland may be underactive. Read the statements below, decide on the level of severity or frequency of each sign or symptom, and then circle the number that most accurately reflects how that statement applies to you:

0 = None or never   1 = Mild or occasionally

2 = Moderate or often   3 = Severe or always

At the bottom of each page, total up the points circled and write the page total. Carry these totals forward to the end of the section. Multiply the number of points in the first section by 2, then add the points from the second section to come up with a grand total.

Section 1

0   1   2   3   My knees are weak or stiff.

0   1   2   3   My back or leg aches.

0   1   2   3   I've been diagnosed with fibromyalgia.

0   1   2   3   I've been diagnosed with carpal tunnel syndrome.

0   1   2   3   I get strange sounds in my ears: ringing, buzzing, clicking, or rumbling, or sounds of running water.

0   1   2   3   I have chronic constipation.

0   1   2   3   I've been losing a lot of hair.

0   1   2   3   I rarely perspire, no matter how hot it is or even if I'm exercising.

0   1   2   3   My heart appears enlarged on an X-ray.

0   1   2   3   I've been diagnosed with chronic fatigue syndrome.

0   1   2   3   The ends of my eyebrows (toward my temples) are getting much thinner and shorter.

0   1   2   3   I have deep-seated pain between my shoulder blades.

0   1   2   3   I have grooves on my fingernails.

0   1   2   3   I have a lot of aches and pains in my joints, hands, or feet.

0   1   2   3   I get a lot of sinus infections.

Page total: _____

0   1   2   3   My tongue seems to be getting bigger, and the sides of it are rippled from pressing against my teeth.

0   1   2   3   My voice is hoarse or weak a lot of the time.

0   1   2   3   I feel uncoordinated and have a tendency to fall for no reason.

0   1   2   3   I've started to talk very slowly, haltingly, and in a monotone.

0   1   2   3   I have a skin disorder such as psoriasis, eczema, or vitiligo.

0   1   2   3   I have ADHD (attention-deficit/hyperactivity disorder).

0   1   2   3   I have gout.

0   1   2   3   My neck is thickening or bulging in the front under my Adam's apple.

0   1   2   3   I sometimes have visual hallucinations such as small animals running across the room.

0   1   2   3   I have an autoimmune disease such as Crohn's disease, sarcoidosis, lupus, multiple sclerosis, scleroderma, rheumatoid arthritis, Sjögren's syndrome, diabetes, or myasthenia gravis.

0   1   2   3   I have Raynaud's syndrome.

0   1   2   3   I have emphysema.

0   1   2   3   I've had a hysterectomy.

0   1   2   3   I've been diagnosed with atherosclerosis (heart disease).

Total number of points for section 1: _____

Total number of points for section 1: _____ x 2 = _____

Section 2

0   1   2   3   My fingernails are soft and thin, and they crack and break easily.

0   1   2   3   I produce a lot of tartar on my teeth and have to have them cleaned often.

0   1   2   3   My neck often gets stiff.

0   1   2   3   I've started to have very heavy periods.

0   1   2   3   I'm gaining weight and neither diet nor exercise seems to control it.

0   1   2   3   I'm losing my eyelashes.

0   1   2   3   I've developed asthma.

0   1   2   3   My gums bleed easily or get red and swollen and have started to recede.

Section 2 page total: _____

0	1	2	3	I've had one or more miscarriages.
0	1	2	3	I'm getting fine wrinkles on my face and hands.
0	1	2	3	I sometimes feel as though bugs are crawling on my skin.
0	1	2	3	I sometimes get burning sensations in various parts of my body.
0	1	2	3	I have ingrown toenails or fungal infections of my toes.
0	1	2	3	I have problems with night vision.
0	1	2	3	I get dizzy sometimes or have been told I have vertigo.
0	1	2	3	I've developed knock-knees.
0	1	2	3	I get sprains easily.
0	1	2	3	My stomach is distended and I have a lot of gas.
0	1	2	3	I have a drinking or substance abuse problem.
0	1	2	3	I smoke cigarettes.
0	1	2	3	I don't tolerate alcohol well.
0	1	2	3	I have hypoglycemia.
0	1	2	3	I have swollen eyelids or swelling under my eyes.
0	1	2	3	My lips are pale.
0	1	2	3	I find myself clenching my teeth often, especially at night.
0	1	2	3	I find myself tapping my foot or jiggling my leg often.
0	1	2	3	I've been diagnosed with temporomandibular joint syndrome.
0	1	2	3	I get recurrent ear infections.
0	1	2	3	I have a lot of dental problems, including getting new cavities.
0	1	2	3	I've developed allergies.
0	1	2	3	I'm easily fatigued.
0	1	2	3	I have slow reflexes.
0	1	2	3	I get very depressed in the winter.
0	1	2	3	My lips appear swollen.
0	1	2	3	I've been diagnosed with sciatica.
0	1	2	3	I have prematurely gray hair.

Page total: _____

0	I	2	3	The skin on my legs is rough or scaly, particularly below my knees.
0	I	2	3	I have anemia.
0	I	2	3	I have diabetes.
0	I	2	3	My face is pale.
0	I	2	3	My hair is dry and brittle.
0	I	2	3	I have a lot of earwax.
0	I	2	3	I don't seem to be able to control my rage and fury, and sometimes I lash out at people.
0	I	2	3	I have a lot of moles and warts.
0	I	2	3	I have elevated LDL cholesterol and/or low HDL cholesterol.
0	I	2	3	My feet are getting flatter.
0	I	2	3	I have fibrocystic breasts and they get very tender and sore.
0	I	2	3	Sex doesn't interest me anymore.
0	I	2	3	I get very irritable and moody.
0	I	2	3	I'm almost always tired no matter how much sleep or rest I get.
0	I	2	3	My thoughts are getting strange.
0	I	2	3	I'm often anxious or agitated.
0	I	2	3	I get a lot of headaches.
0	I	2	3	My hands and feet feel swollen and it isn't due to weight gain.
0	I	2	3	My blood pressure is too high or too low.
0	I	2	3	Simple things have become confusing and sometimes overwhelming.
0	I	2	3	My PMS symptoms are getting worse.
0	I	2	3	I have a hard time concentrating much of the time.
0	I	2	3	I'm having a hard time getting pregnant or had a hard time getting pregnant.
0	I	2	3	My hands and feet get tingling pins-and-needles feelings.
0	I	2	3	I've started to get acne.
0	I	2	3	I have flaky, red patches on my face.
0	I	2	3	I look older than my age.

Page total: _____

0	I	2	3	I have a hard time falling asleep at night.
0	I	2	3	I've been feeling very sad or depressed.
0	I	2	3	I seem to get sick a lot and have a hard time bouncing back.
0	I	2	3	I have restless legs at night.
0	I	2	3	I have heart palpitations and skipped heartbeats.
0	I	2	3	It sometimes feels as though I'm having a heart attack or panic attack.
0	I	2	3	I feel like I'm going crazy sometimes.
0	I	2	3	I've had an abnormal Pap test or have been diagnosed with cervical dysplasia.
0	I	2	3	My skin has an overall puffy or "quilted" look; even my back looks puffy.
0	I	2	3	My hands and feet are always cold.
0	I	2	3	I'm extremely bothered by heat and/or cold.
0	I	2	3	I seem to have almost no body hair anymore.
0	I	2	3	I have hemorrhoids.
0	I	2	3	I have a chronically low basal body temperature when measured with a thermometer.
0	I	2	3	I bruise easily.
0	I	2	3	I get frequent urinary tract or bladder infections.
0	I	2	3	I have a weak, soft pulse.
0	I	2	3	My face and eyelids are puffy.
0	I	2	3	I have incredibly dry skin, especially on my feet.
0	I	2	3	My vision has become variable and is sometimes blurry or shaky.
0	I	2	3	Sometimes I can't hear well out of one or both ears.
0	I	2	3	My skin is yellowish and pale or the whites of my eyes are yellowish.
0	I	2	3	I'm often breathless, and it's hard to catch my breath even when I'm not exerting myself.
0	I	2	3	The skin on my upper arms and the front of my thighs appears to be getting thicker when I pinch it.
0	I	2	3	My urine is scant and often brightly colored.
0	I	2	3	I've started to have irregular menstrual cycles.

Page total: _____

0	1	2	3	I have dyslexia.
0	1	2	3	I'm left-handed.
0	1	2	3	I have mitral valve prolapse.
0	1	2	3	I have ulcerative colitis.
0	1	2	3	I have tendinitis.
0	1	2	3	I've lost my appetite and often food doesn't appeal to me.
0	1	2	3	I've started to choke on small objects or have choking sensations.
0	1	2	3	My face has taken on a masklike, expressionless look.
0	1	2	3	Any wounds I get are very slow to heal.
0	1	2	3	I have a lot of nasal congestion.
0	1	2	3	I have nightmares or strange dreams.
0	1	2	3	I started my menstrual periods before age ten or after age fifteen.
0	1	2	3	My nail beds are pale.
0	1	2	3	I've had pneumonia.
0	1	2	3	I find myself yawning a lot.
0	1	2	3	I have varicose veins.
0	1	2	3	I've been diagnosed with a frozen shoulder.

Section 2 page total: _____

Total number of points for section 2: _____

Total number of points for section 1: _____

Total number of points: _____

Interpreting Your Results

If your total is between 10 and 15, you're beginning to show signs of possible hypothyroidism; if your total is between 16 and 21 your deficiency is getting more serious. If your score is over 22, you're most likely experiencing significant thyroid function deficiency (and possibly adrenal imbalance as well). With any of these results, you should have a complete physical, including a thyroid exam and lab tests to measure blood levels of free T3, free T4, TSH, and reverse T3, as well as thyroid antibodies if your doctor feels it's warranted. (See chapter 6 for more on these tests.) Since your thyroid is affected by your other endocrine glands, it is also important to measure levels of FSH, estrogen, progesterone, testosterone, DHEA (dehydroepiandrosterone) , and cortisol.

EXERCISE: Hyperthyroidism Symptom Evaluation

This test will help you determine whether you may have an overactive thyroid gland. Read the statements below, decide on the level of severity or frequency of each sign or symptom, and then circle the number that most accurately reflects how that statement applies to you:

0 = None or never

1 = Mild or occasionally

2 = Moderate or often

3 = Severe or always

At the bottom of the list, total up the points circled to get a final score.

0 1 2 3   I've been having more bowel movements than usual.

0 1 2 3   My hands tremble a lot for no reason.

0 1 2 3   My skin has been unusually warm and moist.

0 1 2 3   I've been losing weight even though I haven't cut back on what I eat.

0 1 2 3   My eyes have begun to look as if I'm staring all the time and even seem to be bugging out or protruding.

0 1 2 3   My eyes have become red and irritated for no reason.

0 1 2 3   I have become noticeably more nervous and agitated.

0 1 2 3   The skin on my lower legs seem to be thickening.

0 1 2 3   I have insomnia.

0 1 2 3   I feel overheated a lot of the time.

0 1 2 3   I feel wired but tired a lot of the time.

0 1 2 3   My breathing is more rapid than usual, and sometimes I have a hard time catching my breath.

0 1 2 3   I get very irritable for no reason.

0 1 2 3   My muscles feel very weak sometimes.

Total number of points: _____

Interpreting Your Results

If your total points are between 8 and 12, you're beginning to show signs of possible hyperthyroidism; if your total is between 13 and 18 your condition is more serious. If your score is over 18, you're most likely experiencing significant hyperthyroidism. With any of these results, you should have a complete physical, including a thyroid exam and lab tests to measure blood levels of free T3, free T4, and TSH, as well as thyroid antibodies. (See chapter 6 for more on these tests.) See chapter 11 for full details on hyperthyroidism.

TESTS YOU CAN DO AT HOME

If either symptom evaluation indicated that you may have thyroid dysfunction, the next step is to see your doctor and have lab tests of various hormone levels. In the meanwhile, here are some easy and inexpensive tests you can do at home first. Although these tests aren't definitive, they will give you additional helpful information that you can take to your doctor visit. Many doctors who specialize in thyroid treatment ask their patients to start with the basal thermometer test as an indicator of metabolic rate. If this test reveals chronic low basal body temperature, they'll often prescribe a trial treatment with thyroid hormones.

Basal Body Temperature Test

Your basal body temperature can be used to gauge your thyroid's ability to regulate your body temperature. When you're healthy, you have a very consistent temperature of about 98.4°F. A temperature that drops below 97.8°F is too low and is a red flag for low thyroid function or a low metabolic rate. A reading above 98.4°F may indicate hyperthyroidism.

Most doctors recommend that you do this simple test for ten days in a row. If you still have a period, begin on day one of your period; otherwise you can do it anytime.

1. The night before testing, shake down a glass basal thermometer to below 95°F.

2. The next morning, as soon as you wake up and before you get out of bed, put the thermometer under your arm with the bulb in your armpit.

3. Lie still for ten minutes.

4. Remove the thermometer, read it, and record your results.

5. Do this test every morning for the next ten days.

A normal reading falls between 97.8°F and 98.4°F. If yours is below this range, you have an increased probability of hypothyroidism. If it's higher, you may have hyperthyroidism or a low-grade infection.

Iodine Deficiency Test for Hypothyroidism

Iodine is essential for your thyroid gland to produce thyroid hormones. Without enough iodine in your diet, conversion of T4 to T3 is decreased, which can eventually lead to hypothyroidism. This helps explain why many people don't respond well to thyroid supplementation. Try this test to see if an iodine deficiency might be causing your thyroid problem:

1. Buy 2 percent tincture of iodine at the drugstore.

2. With the applicator or a cotton swab, apply a patch of iodine the size of a quarter on your stomach or thigh.

3. Watch the spot periodically for the next twenty-four hours. If it disappears in less than twenty-four hours, it indicates iodine deficiency. The faster it disappears, the greater the deficiency.

If you don't use much salt, or if you use non-iodized salt, you may be deficient in iodine. If so, you need to either use more salt or take an iodine supplement.

Pinch Test for Myxedema Due to Hypothyroidism

A simple pinch test can indicate whether you have *myxedema*, a common symptom of hypothyroidism. This condition results in swelling due to low metabolic activity and the resulting buildup of wastes in the tissues. Myxedema is most commonly seen in areas such as the face (above and below the eyes and on the jawline) and the front of the upper arms and legs.

Simply pinch a fold of skin on the inside of your upper arm (toward the body) between your thumb and forefinger. If it feels thick and it's hard to pinch a small amount of skin, you most likely have some level of myxedema.

Swallow Test

The swallow test detects swelling of your thyroid (a goiter) or possibly a nodule on your thyroid. These conditions may be caused by either hypothyroidism or hyperthyroidism. This easy self-exam requires nothing more than a mirror and a glass of water.

Simply look at the base of the front of your neck (between your Adam's apple and your collarbone) in a mirror. Then tip your head back and swallow a mouthful of water. As you swallow, note any bulging or protrusion around your thyroid. Repeat this several times until you're sure whether or not you see a bulge. If you do notice a bulge, you may have a thyroid problem.

WHAT'S NEXT?

Now that you've completed the symptom evaluations and tried the simple home tests, you should have a much better idea of the status of your thyroid function. If your responses indicate potential problems with your thyroid function, schedule an appointment with your doctor as soon as possible so that you can have your thyroid examined and your levels of thyroid hormones tested. Armed with the results, you can start working on solutions. (As you'll learn in chapter 6, it's important to work with a doctor experienced in thyroid and endocrine health.)

The information you got from the symptom evaluations in this chapter is the most valuable tool your doctor will have for accurately diagnosing and treating your thyroid situation, since thyroid testing is an inexact science. (As you'll learn in chapter 6, you may have thyroid dysfunction even if your thyroid hormone levels are in the "normal" ranges.) Take a copy of your symptom evaluation with you to your doctor's appointment. Doctors often have to try to piece together what's going on with incomplete or even inaccurate data. The work you've done here will give your doctor a comprehensive overview of your symptoms.

Since you may have to wait a while for a doctor's appointment, in the meanwhile you can continue working your way through this book. If your evaluation indicated possible hypothyroidism, turn to the next chapter to learn more about your symptoms and what they mean. If you think you may have hyperthyroidism, turn to chapter 11. In either case, continue to observe your symptoms so that you can provide your doctor with detailed, accurate information.

KEY POINTS

🗶 Thyroid dysfunction affects every organ and gland in your body, and therefore manifests in a myriad of diverse symptoms. These symptoms are valuable indicators of what's going on with your thyroid function.

🗶 To truly understand your thyroid health, it's vital to inventory and assess your symptoms. Thyroid testing is valuable, but a complete understanding of thyroid status is only possible when testing is combined with a comprehensive analysis of your symptoms.

🗶 Several easy, inexpensive home tests may be done to further evaluate your thyroid function before you go to see your doctor. They include the basal body temperature test, the iodine deficiency test, the pinch test for myxedema, and the swallow test.

CHAPTER 4

Understanding Symptoms of Hypothyroidism

The things that can go wrong with your body when your thyroid function is low are so pervasive and extensive it's startling. So many of the difficulties and indignities we learn to live with, thinking they're an inevitable part of aging, are actually the result of low thyroid function and are reversible. As you read this chapter, you may find it hard to believe that your thyroid can have such powerful effects throughout your body. But the truth of the matter is that adequate thyroid function plays an important role in maintaining good quality of life as we age and staying free from pain and disease. Our basic bodily functions, general well-being, appearance, energy levels, mental function, emotions, and even our very sanity all depend on adequate thyroid function. Because symptoms that affect physical appearance often show up initially (and can be so distressing), let's look at them first.

PHYSICAL APPEARANCE

As we age, we certainly want to take advantage of everything that can keep us youthful, attractive, and svelte. Who needs plastic surgery when maintaining good thyroid function is a cheap, noninvasive way to stave off accelerated aging? When you take a close look at the impact low thyroid function can have on all parts of your body, you'll realize that you need to take your thyroid seriously in order to age gracefully.

Hair

Since hair and skin are some of our fastest growing tissues, we often notice slowing metabolism in these areas first. Hypothyroidism leads to hair that is dry, brittle, and dull. It also becomes straighter, finer, and thinner and may even turn gray prematurely. Thin, uneven, patchy gray hair isn't the look we're after as we head into our forties or fifties! Another sign of low thyroid function, discovered over a century ago, is the loss of the outer third of the eyebrows. Body hair and eyelashes also often disappear.

Skin

Slowing thyroid function takes a big toll on the skin. The first signs are coarse, dry, sallow, pale, unhealthy looking skin, which also may get very itchy (Owen and Lazarus 2003). This can progress to acne, red spots, boils, premature wrinkling, yellowing or grayish skin, rashes, and even eczema or psoriasis. Adequate thyroid function is necessary for good blood circulation, so hypothyroidism results in inadequate blood flow throughout your body. When this happens, blood is preferentially sent to your brain and vital organs to keep essential functions going. Our skin may be our largest organ, but in hypothyroidism it takes a backseat to survival, and as a result, it isn't properly nourished and replenished by the oxygen that blood provides. Poor circulation can also lead to the development of varicose veins.

Skin can also get puffy and swollen, particularly on the face, arms, and front of the thighs due to fluid building up in the connective tissues. This condition, known as myxedema, is a side effect of slowed metabolism. It's caused by an accumulation of waste products that aren't effectively removed from the tissues. Connective tissue is everywhere in the body, so this swelling doesn't affect just physical appearance; it also impacts the function of the glands, organs, and cells as they become infiltrated with this jellylike substance. In fact, this swelling may affect only internal tissues and organs, without showing any external signs.

Face

When thyroid function is low, the face, particularly around the eyes and jawline, often gets puffy; this, too, is caused by myxedema. Reduced kidney function caused by the general slowing of metabolism also leads to fluid retention, particularly around the eyes and in the hands and ankles. This is a different type of edema and can be distinguished from myxedema by pressing your finger on it; if it leaves a depression that lasts for a longer period of time than is normal, it's due to reduced kidney function rather than myxedema. As hypothyroidism progresses, the entire face can develop a coarse look, with swelling or thickening of facial features.

Fingernails and Toenails

Slow-growing, soft, ridged, brittle nails with pale nail beds are a sign of low thyroid function. The crescent-shaped white area at the base of the nail bed often gets lighter or disappears altogether. This can be due to reduced blood circulation or inadequate protein synthesis, another effect of the general slowing of metabolism in hypothyroidism (Jabbour 2003). Ingrown toenails and fungal infections are also common.

Teeth and Mouth

Excessive tartar buildup and cavities can be caused by low thyroid function (Noren and Alm 1983). Excess tarter causes red, swollen, and receding gums (which can be made worse by low estrogen), hence the old saying "getting long in the tooth." Gum recession isn't always a reliable sign of hypothyroidism, however, as gum disease due to hypothyroidism can also cause gums to become swollen and overdeveloped and extend down over the teeth instead of receding.

In long-standing hypothyroidism, the mouth can appear large and the lips puffy and coarse. The color inside the mouth is often pale, and the palate may be more vaulted than usual (Barker, Hoskins, and Mosenthal 1922). Temporomandibular joint syndrome (TMJ syndrome) is also common as hypothyroidism causes problems with muscles and ligaments. In addition, both edema and clenched teeth due to chronic muscular tension can affect the jaw and cause the pain and muscle spasms of TMJ syndrome.

Weight

With hypothyroidism, we don't metabolize food effectively and the calories we consume turn into fat instead of energy. This weight gain is insidious, and neither diet nor exercise resolves it. When weight gain is caused strictly by low thyroid function and not other endocrine deficiencies as well, fat tends to be symmetrically distributed on the body (Barker, Hoskins, and Mosenthal 1922). When low pituitary function is at the root of low thyroid function, weight gain is generally confined to the area from your abdomen to just above your knees. The skin of a person with hypothyroidism also takes on a flabby look, as overall musculature is affected, too. Bear in mind that being overweight is an issue that goes beyond mere appearances, as it increases your risk of many diseases and health conditions.

Feet and Legs

Do you have weak knees, or have you become flat-footed or bowlegged in recent years? All of the ligaments in your body can be affected by low thyroid function. They will tend to relax and can cause conditions like flat feet, weak knees, knock-knees, hyperflexibility of joints, propensity for sprains, and even scoliosis. Early on in hypothyroidism, the knees often get weak. This starts with a feeling of unreliability in the knees, as if your knees might give out if you were to break into a jog or even a fast walk.

The first sign that your ligaments are being affected is often a flattening of the arches of your feet. When they flatten, your foot rotates inward, which can result in painful calluses on the sides of your big toes and sore, aching feet. Another sign of relaxing ligaments is aching palms (Jacobs-Kosmin and DeHoratius 2005).

Voice

Although it can't be seen, the voice is an obvious indicator of age and health. Due to swelling in the throat, many women with hypothyroidism start to sound more weak and tired. The voice often gets deeper and softer and also more hoarse or nasal. Speech can become deliberate and slow, and as the condition progresses, articulating words may become difficult, causing stumbling over words and slurred speech (Madariaga et al. 2002). These difficulties can stem from swelling of the lips and tongue.

As with being overweight, changes to the voice have impacts beyond the impression you make on others. The swelling of the throat responsible for voice changes also causes difficulties with swallowing, so choking on small objects is common. If the uvula (the little punching bag in the back of your throat) and tonsils swell, this can cause snoring and an inability to breath through the nose.

Ears

Not only does low thyroid function result in chronic ear infections due to lowered immune function, it can also result in impaired hearing and abnormal physical ear placement. If long-standing, hypothyroidism can cause the ears can be set lower on the head and protrude more, while also becoming more swollen or thicker than normal. Overall hearing is diminished and excessive earwax is common (Brucker-Davis et al. 1996). Low thyroid function can also cause tinnitus and result in hearing strange noises, such as clicking, ringing, or buzzing sounds or the sound of running water.

Posture

As our thyroid function declines, so does our ability to hold ourselves upright. Posture is one of the markers of aging, with stooped and slumped posture being part and parcel of the look of old women. Poor posture may be caused by the fatigue so common in hypothyroidism, or by the bone weakening and osteoporosis that also occur. This slumping is exacerbated when the abdomen protrudes due to relaxing musculature and swelling of the stomach caused by constipation.

Musculature

Few things signal aging more than flabby, diminishing muscles. Our muscles are closely tied to the metabolic process, and when it slows, they start to lose their tone and contours. The weight gain we experience at the same time obscures them even more. But again, this goes beyond appearances. Normal activities will become more difficult as the muscles also get tired easily and often feel heavy, and mobility can be impaired by an increased tendency to stumble or experience muscle cramps (Argov et al. 1988).

Donna's Story

Donna was forty-two when she first felt she was losing the battle to aging. She had been fine up to that point; although she had gained a few pounds, she wasn't overly concerned. She remembered what her mother had always told her: that women should gain ten pounds every decade in order to keep their youthful figures and have their skin remain plump and firm. She had always figured she was in that range, as up to age forty, she had only gained fifteen pounds since her midtwenties, when she had her first child.

Unfortunately, she had recently gained an additional ten pounds and wasn't looking rounded and firm anymore, but rather more lumpy and sagging. It seemed that no matter what she ate her weight continued to creep up. She even tried a three-day fast, to no avail. She also started to have trouble with her feet. They ached a lot of the time and she had developed painful calluses on the outside edges of her big toes. She went to an podiatrist for help, but he told her that this was an inevitable part of aging and that the only solution was to get orthotics for her shoes, as the calluses meant she was getting flat feet, making her feet rotate inward. He fitted her for the orthotics and sure enough, as soon as she started to wear them, her calluses went away and her feet stopped hurting. Unfortunately, this ruled out most of her fashionable shoes, but she didn't have any alternatives given the discomfort.

At the same time, her knees started to get very weak and tended to buckle when she climbed stairs or walked quickly. This, coupled with an ever-increasing tendency to slump, made her feel like an old lady. Back to the doctor she went, this time an orthopedist. He took X-rays of her knees and said that she had some cartilage damage in her right knee and should consider getting fitted for a leg brace. She'd had a skiing accident twenty years before, which probably accounted for the damage, but as it had never caused her any problem she couldn't imagine that this was what was causing the weakness. And the thought of a brace on top of the orthotics was too much, so she decided she would just have to live with the weakness and be careful when she walked fast.

What finally got her to consider that something serious might be going on was when her hair started to fall out. This was too much—she could hardly bear to look at herself in the mirror anymore. Between the weight gain, her slumped posture, her thinning hair, and those horrible shoes, it was time to do something, so she scheduled an appointment with her doctor.

Donna was delighted with her appointment. She had pessimistically feared that it was all in her mind; simply a matter of willpower, or not working out enough, or something else that she just wasn't doing right. Her doctor surprised her by saying that she had many signs of low thyroid function and that a few simple tests should get to the bottom of the situation.

When she returned to get her tests results, her doctor told her that all her tests indicated low thyroid function and that supplemental thyroid hormones should make a huge difference in how she was feeling. She started on thyroid hormone therapy and almost immediately felt much stronger. Her knees stopped giving out, and slowly but surely the weight started to come off. After about three months, she realized that the calluses didn't come back when she wore her regular shoes, so she was able to give up the orthotics. At about the same time, she also noticed her hair was regaining its former thickness and shine. It was as if she had rolled the clock back ten years!

THE MIND AND EMOTIONS

It isn't just our physical appearance that is negatively affected by low thyroid hormone levels; our minds suffer just as many discouraging side effects. These effects can be subtle and hard to recognize, as with low-grade depression, which may show up as fatigue or lack of interest in activities that we used to enjoy. But mental and emotional effects can also be extreme. In severe cases, people may experience hallucinations and delusions, such as hearing voices or ringing bells, or seeing small scampering animals. In fact, in the early part of the twentieth century, Nelson W. Janney, MD, described "a type of hypothyroid insanity occurring in women about menopause," with symptoms of "mental confusion, loss of memory, and delusions of persecution" (Janney 1922, 411). How many of us fit into this category?

Psychological Health

Emotional stability can be severely compromised by low thyroid function. There are more T3 receptors in the brain than anywhere else in the body, and when these receptors don't get enough T3 thyroid hormone stimulation, the effect on the brain can impact our emotional stability profoundly. This can show up in many ways, the most common being depression, which is becoming frighteningly common. Research has shown that about twenty million people in the United States suffer from depression. That's one in ten adults (National Institute of Mental Health 2008), and women are about twice as likely as men to be affected (Substance Abuse and Mental Health Services Administration 2005).

Although antidepressant drugs can provide a short-term solution, they don't fix the underlying problem and also leave most women feeling somewhat detached. Although they no longer experience the uncontrollable anger and sadness they did before starting on antidepressants, they also don't feel emotions as strongly and may derive less enjoyment from life. Of even greater concern is that fluoxetine (Prozac), one of the most common antidepressant drugs, contains fluorine, which is known to suppress thyroid function, thereby exacerbating the underlying situation if thyroid dysfunction plays a role in the depression.

We can also get very irritable and anxious when our thyroid hormone levels drop, and even become downright hostile and angry. Contrary to what our partner, friends, and family think, this is something we often can't control. Despite our best intentions of controlling our temper and not letting things get to us, our overstressed nervous systems are easily triggered and we lash out at seemingly trivial things. When irritability and anxiety are caused by low thyroid hormone levels, the only cure is to restore healthy thyroid function. With proper thyroid treatment, the anger, hostility, and anxiety all disappear quickly.

Social isolation is also a common symptom of hypothyroidism. Women suffering from hypothyroidism may withdraw from relationships because they feel their friends no longer like them or that they're critical. They may find themselves losing long-term friends one by one and giving up the social activities they used to enjoy. Many other mental conditions, some of them very serious, can also be caused by low thyroid hormone levels, including bipolar disorder, schizophrenia, senility, and even paranoid psychosis (Greenspan and Gardner 2000).

Memory and Cognitive Ability

Optimal levels of thyroid hormones are required for our minds to process information and work as they should. There are basic biological differences between our brains and those of men that make us more subject to cognitive troubles when our thyroid isn't functioning properly. Women have fewer brain cells than men do, but each of these brain cells has far more connections to other parts of the brain than men's brain cells do (Rabinowicz et al. 1999). This allows us to use more areas of our brain at the same time, which results in enhanced brain function. The increased demand of this larger network requires more energy and greater blood flow. Thyroid hormones, as well as estrogen, are required for optimum blood flow, so low thyroid hormone levels cause an actual decrease in brain function (Owen and Lazarus 2003). This is why we lose our ability to concentrate in that aptly named condition known as brain fog. It also results in memory loss and decreased ability for deductive reasoning. Things that we used to be able to figure out easily may become confusing and seemingly more complex.

BASIC BODILY FUNCTIONS

All of our basic bodily functions are affected by the thyroid. Our metabolic rate, driven by thyroid hormones, determines whether things run smoothly and optimally or slowly and inefficiently. Everything from blood pressure and breathing to digestion and nerve function can by impacted by thyroid dysfunction, and the effects can be profound.

od Pressure

bnormal blood pressure (most often low but sometimes high) is common in hypothyroidism. As roid hormone levels start to drop, low blood pressure usually develops. Ongoing low thyroid function results in inadequate kidney function, which can ultimately trigger the body to increase blood pressure in an attempt to force more blood through the kidneys to increase their filtering rate. This process is progressive and can result in ever-increasing blood pressure. At the same time, increasing cholesterol (also caused by hypothyroidism) is narrowing the arteries, requiring the heart to pump harder to get blood through them. Hypothyroidism is associated with increases in diastolic blood pressure (the bottom measurement). A common finding is a decreasing difference between the top and bottom measurements as the top reading gets lower and the bottom reading gets higher (Kahaly and Dillmann 2005).

The blood itself generally has reduced numbers of red blood cells, causing a reduction in oxygenation and an increase in carbon dioxide levels throughout the body. Anemia may also result. Low white blood cell count is also common, which impairs your body's overall immune function and ability to fight infections. These abnormal red and white blood cell counts can be seen on standard blood tests.

Body Temperature

Intolerance of heat and cold is the norm with low thyroid function. We feel better when it's warm but get acutely uncomfortable when it's hot. Body temperature directly reflects metabolic rate so if your body temperature is low (as measured by a basal thermometer), then your metabolic rate is as well. Inability to perspire is also a common symptom, as the body isn't able to effectively regulate its temperature without adequate thyroid function (Silva 1995).

Fluid Retention

Hypothyroidism results in fluid retention. There are two types of fluid retention that plague women with low thyroid function. The first is that caused by myxedema, where waste products that build up over time are held in a chemical matrix in the tissues. This condition doesn't respond to diuretics. The only way to get rid of this condition is to increase thyroid hormone levels, which allows the trapped fluid to be released. However, it often takes some time on thyroid hormone therapy to resolve the problem.

The second type of fluid retention is caused when hypothyroidism reduces kidney function, resulting in inadequate blood filtration and fluid balance. The net physical effect of this process is puffiness in the hands, ankles, and face, particularly around the eyes. This kind of edema, which leaves a depression when you press a finger against the affected area, does respond to diuretics.

Digestion and Elimination

Constipation is extremely common in hypothyroidism as both digestion of food and excretion of wastes are slowed, along with everything else in the body. The specific cause is deficient muscular action of the abdominal walls and intestines. Nerves and muscles are critical in the lengthy process of digestion, in which food must navigate almost thirty feet of intestines. When nerve and muscle function are slowed by low thyroid function, this process is slowed as well. The normal time between eating and a bowel movement varies from woman to woman, but is usually between twelve and thirty-six hours. With hypothyroidism, this process can take much longer—in some cases up to a week. This results in painful bowel movements and hemorrhoids, as well as a buildup of toxins as waste products are not excreted as they should be. The fermentation of wastes caused by the extended time it takes for food to move through your digestive tract often results in large quantities of gas, which distends the abdomen.

In addition, production of digestive enzymes and gastric acid is reduced, impairing your body's ability to properly digest and utilize nutrients. Excretion of liquid waste is affected, too. Hypothyroidism has a profound effect on the bladder, causing less urine to be produced. It also causes the lining of the bladder to be easily irritated, resulting in frequent and painful urination and bladder infections.

Heart Health

Heart disease is the number one cause of death for women in the United States, and the biggest threat to heart health as we age is atherosclerosis (American Heart Association 2008). This condition develops silently and insidiously as LDL (bad cholesterol) is deposited along artery walls, causing them to narrow. High LDL levels aren't caused by diet alone, as a significant amount of cholesterol is made in the body, not consumed. Because low thyroid function affects your body's ability to process fats properly, it can contribute to excessive production of LDL cholesterol. This condition is exacerbated by the low liver function common in hypothyroidism, which slows the metabolism and excretion of excess cholesterol.

The heart muscle itself is weakened when not stimulated by adequate thyroid hormones, causing the heart to work harder and actually enlarge in size, which can be seen if the heart is X-rayed. This weakening of the heart causes symptoms such as heart palpitations, angina, breathlessness, and fluid retention and can ultimately result in congestive heart failure (Kahaly and Dillmann 2005). The pulse rate is usually slower in hypothyroidism, too, causing sluggish circulation.

Breathing

With hypothyroidism, breathing becomes shallow and slow, and it becomes harder and harder to take deep breaths. Asthma also becomes more common. Many people have a sensation of "air hunger," or not being able to get enough air. One reason for this is loss of tone in the muscles involved in breathing; another is nervous system problems that cause inadequate signaling to those muscles.

Nerve Function

Our nerves suffer when surrounding tissues and blood vessels, which help keep them healthy, are compromised by slowed circulation and the resulting oxygen deficiency. Strange sensations can result, including numbness, burning, tingling, and, the strangest one of all, the feeling of bugs crawling on the skin. Two common nervous system conditions rarely recognized as symptoms of low thyroid function are carpal tunnel syndrome and restless legs syndrome (RLS). Low thyroid function can cause carpal tunnel syndrome due to swelling that compresses the median nerve in the wrist. In fact, a new study suggests that this condition isn't caused by repetitive motion, such as computer keyboard use, as has been generally believed (Atroshi et al. 2007). Research on restless legs syndrome has indicated there may be a link between thyroid disorders and RLS, but no conclusive evidence is available yet. Estimates suggest that approximately 25 percent of all cases of RLS are caused by anemia, so anemia due to hypothyroidism may be at the root of these cases. Further, studies have shown that when people with thyroid disorders experience symptoms similar to RLS, those symptoms may improve or resolve with thyroid treatment (Tan et al. 2005).

Liver Function

Deficient liver function is common in hypothyroidism. When it's significant it causes elevated liver enzymes on lab tests, but usually it goes undetected. This can cause a grave threat to your health, as your liver is responsible for performing an astonishingly large number of tasks that impact all systems in your body. Thyroid hormones act as metabolic stimulants and increase the rate of oxygen consumption by the liver. Without proper stimulation, the liver becomes sluggish and can't properly do its job of filtering harmful substances from the blood, breaking down fats, storing vitamins and minerals, producing urea, making amino acids for the production of proteins, and maintaining a proper level of glucose in the blood. The liver also produces cholesterol, which is needed for many critical functions such as making hormones, and is also responsible for metabolizing and excreting cholesterol to keep levels from getting too high (Bayraktar and van Thiel 1997). Since the liver is responsible for ensuring constant blood sugar levels, low liver function can lead to *hypoglycemia*, which simply means low blood sugar. Hypoglycemia results in headaches, as well as feeling shaky, anxious, weak, and tired.

Mobility

Decreased mobility is the norm in hypothyroidism due to myxedema, in which waste-laden fluids build up in muscles, ligaments, and other tissues. In effect, the entire body can become swollen, stiff, and weak, compromising mobility and sometimes coordination and balance. When this condition progresses, it can affect your ability to walk and cause balance problems, including stumbling and falling. In addition, dizziness and vertigo, which are also symptoms of low thyroid function, can exacerbate problems with balance and mobility.

Sleep

Insomnia and sleep apnea are common in hypothyroidism. Because of the thickening and swelling of the nasal mucous passages due to myxedema, snoring, snuffling, and mouth breathing are also common, as are sinus infections and other respiratory infections, which can interfere with a good night's sleep. Low thyroid function usually results in having a very hard time getting to sleep, while low estrogen levels result in a light, disturbed sleep, where you wake up several times during the night.

Eyesight

Eyesight is also almost always affected by hypothyroidism. Conditions related to low thyroid function include visual disturbances, loss of acuity, night-blindness, and even glaucoma and cataracts (Gawaii et al. 2003). There are several reasons for this, most notably the body's inability to convert beta-carotene to vitamin A without adequate thyroid function.

Kelly's Story

Kelly was forty-eight when she had a frightening wake-up call during a routine physical. She went in for her annual physical expecting everything to be fine, as it had been at her last checkup two years earlier. She felt relatively well and wasn't having any obvious health problems other than being more tired than she used to be and having a hard time sleeping. Sometimes she would lie in bed for three or four hours before she could fall asleep, leaving her feeling groggy and disoriented most of the next day.

Kelly had also been diagnosed with carpel tunnel syndrome earlier that year and had to wear a splint at night to control the pain and numbness. Her periods had gotten very heavy, and it was hard for her to leave the house for very long on the day of the heaviest flow because she bled so much. However, she figured this was just a temporary condition that would resolve at menopause and wasn't anything to worry about.

Unfortunately, as soon as her doctor entered the exam room frowning, Kelly knew something was wrong. He told her that her blood pressure, which had been creeping up over the last two physicals, was now fairly elevated, and he recommended blood pressure medication. He examined her and told her she seemed fine otherwise, and that he'd call her when he got her lab results back. She took her prescription slip for the blood pressure medication to the pharmacy, worrying about what other problems her blood tests might show.

When her doctor called her with the rest of her results, the news wasn't good. Her bad cholesterol (LDL) was very high, her good cholesterol (HDL) was very low, and her triglycerides were also elevated. He also said that her TSH level was very high, indicating that she needed thyroid medication. She had no idea what her thyroid did so this really worried her.

He told her that he wanted her to start taking thyroid hormones, as well as a statin drug to lower her LDL level. She told him she really didn't want to take any additional drugs, as she had just started on the blood pressure medication and had several unpleasant side effects. He agreed that she could put off starting the statin drug for a couple of months but insisted that she start on the thyroid medication right away.

She started taking the thyroid hormones and the strangest things began to happen. The first thing she noticed was that she started sleeping better almost immediately. She didn't put this together with starting the thyroid medicine until she started to notice other subtle changes as well: Her next period was noticeably lighter for the first time in at least a year, with no more flooding and clotting. Her carpal tunnel symptoms also seemed to be much better, with drastically reduced pain and numbness, and she felt much more cheerful and optimistic than she had in a long time. She even started thinking about maybe getting a part-time job, since her kids were now both in high school. It finally occurred to her that these changes coincided with starting on the thyroid hormones.

The biggest shock came went she went back to the doctor after six months for a follow-up on her blood pressure and cholesterol. Her cholesterol levels were significantly reduced and now in the normal range. When they discussed how this could have happened, her doctor mentioned that he had read several studies that showed that high cholesterol was often tied to low thyroid function, but he admitted that he had never tried thyroid hormone therapy to resolve cholesterol problems (although he now would!). She asked if he would be comfortable with her tapering off her blood pressure medication; since she no longer had a cholesterol problem, maybe they didn't have to worry about heart disease as much. He said that it made sense and agreed that she should give it a try and see what happened. Kelly went back to her doctor when she had been off the medication for a month, and her blood pressure was back to normal!

OVERALL WELL-BEING

It's impossible to be healthy or happy when your thyroid function is too low. You may be able to carry on with daily activities, but your *joie de vivre* disappears, leaving you to slog through one day after another feeling ever more tired and resentful. The things that used to give you pleasure, from simple things like shopping with friends or going to a movie, to the more complex, such as completing a big project at work or a major home improvement project, become progressively more exhausting and draining. Often all you really feel like doing is lying down and doing absolutely nothing.

Energy

It shouldn't come as a surprise that the lowered metabolism found in hypothyroidism would lead to low energy levels; it's just common sense. No organ, tissue, gland, or cell escapes this general slowing. Thyroid hormone supplementation causes the body to increase production of mitochondria, the little energy generators in every one of our cells (Argov et al. 1988). Not only do the numbers of mitochondria increase, their size also increases, allowing them to produce more energy to support the activity of your entire body.

Pain

Widespread and varied pain and stiffness, also called arthralgia, is common in hypothyroidism. It can be caused by muscle fibers separating due to edema and reduced enzyme activity in the muscles (Simonides, van Hardeveld, and Larsen 1992). The buildup of waste products due to myxedema causes a jellylike substance to be deposited in the muscles, ligaments, and joints, causing pain, stiffness, and cramping in the affected areas, most commonly the neck, back, feet, and hands. The back problems that many of us get in perimenopause, which unfortunately are usually treated with corticosteroids like prednisone, are in reality often just a symptom of low thyroid function. The use of these strong anti-inflammatory drugs leads to serious side effects, including osteoporosis, and also inhibits thyroid function, making the problem worse.

Headaches, a very common symptom of hypothyroidism, are also thought to be caused by fluid buildup. Plus, cranial nerves that control many functions in the head, such as hearing, smell, vision, and taste, can be affected. This can cause decreases in these functions and also result in various aches and pains, including headaches and facial pain.

Immune Function

The general slowdown of metabolic activity in hypothyroidism results in the buildup of toxins in our cells, which leads to cell damage and death, affecting our immune function. Plus, when thyroid function is low, resistance to infection is also lowered. Not only do we start catching every cold or flu that's going around, we also have a hard time getting over minor illnesses and may stay sick for weeks instead of days. Our underpowered immune system simply isn't able to respond to these various infections and fight them off as it did in the past.

Among the most common infections for women with low thyroid function are urinary tract infections, which can lead to kidney infections and cystitis when immune function is low. Bladder health in general is dependent on robust levels of thyroid hormones and estrogen. As we lose these key hormones, not only do we get more infections, we also experience problems with urinary frequency and bladder irritability and discomfort. No wonder the going joke among most of us women over fifty (or even forty) is that it's best never to pass up a bathroom opportunity while out shopping with girlfriends, because you never know when you'll need to find one.

51

Other infections common in hypothyroidism are chronic sinus infections, infections of the gastrointestinal tract like colitis, and infections of the musculoskeletal tissue, such as bursitis and tendinitis (which can also be caused by overuse, stress, and direct trauma). Other signs of lowered immune function are slow wound healing and the tendency to pick up every disease we're exposed to.

Autoimmune disease is closely connected with low thyroid function. Diseases such as lupus, rheumatoid arthritis, scleroderma, and polymyositis are characterized by problems with connective tissue. The buildup of fluid in the tissues due to myxedema can have effects that are strikingly similar to the pain and stiffness of these disorders, so if you have one of these diseases, you should have your thyroid function evaluated. Low thyroid function could be having a significant impact on your condition.

Cancer is a complex and intimidating condition. It would be irresponsible to say that good thyroid function can prevent it without an enormous amount of clinical study. However, we do know that the thyroid is responsible for optimal immune function, so the prudent approach to cancer prevention is to optimize your thyroid function and incorporate good dietary and lifestyle practices into your life.

YOUR FEMALE SIDE

Hormonal conditions such as hypothyroidism hit women much harder than men, and the attributes that make us uniquely female are particularly affected. We see changes in everything from our menstrual cycle, to breast development, to libido and fertility. Low thyroid function can often begin at puberty and may cause precocious, or early, puberty or delayed puberty, along with lack of normal menstrual cycle and breast development. Other effects include excessively heavy or prolonged menstrual bleeding, more frequent periods, painful periods that include back and leg aches, nausea, bowel disturbances, and headaches.

Menstrual Cycle

Low thyroid function has a negative effect on our menstrual cycle and results in altered levels of the hormones responsible for causing ovulation. This results in cycles where ovulation doesn't occur, infertility, and the heavy menstrual bleeding so common in perimenopause (Greenspan and Gardner 2000). It can also cause severe cramping and irregular cycles. If you recall that there is a reciprocal relationship between your thyroid and your ovaries, you can see how hypothyroidism can disrupt ovarian function, resulting in low estrogen and progesterone production and ultimately causing irregular ovulation and menstrual periods.

Anemia, which is so common in hypothyroidism, can be caused by iron deficiency due to heavy menstrual periods. However, it may also be due to low levels of red blood cells, impaired synthesis of hemoglobin (the protein in red blood cells that carries oxygen), or low levels of vitamin

B$_{12}$ or folic acid—all of which can also be triggered by low thyroid function. Although low levels of thyroid hormones usually result in early onset of menstruation, in some cases it can delay it as well. If you started your periods before age ten or after age fifteen, this may have been caused by low thyroid function.

Infertility and Miscarriages

Infertility and miscarriages are commonly caused by low thyroid function. The reasons are varied, but one obvious cause of infertility is the failure to ovulate that can result from hypothyroidism. Generally, the risk of miscarriages decreases when thyroid hormone is replaced (Marqusee, Hill, and Mandel 1997), and supplementation may help with infertility, as well, if the infertility is due to hypothyroidism.

Pregnancy and Childbirth

During pregnancy, the thyroid gland goes into overdrive to produce additional thyroid hormones for the baby, so this can be a time of remission from many symptoms of hypothyroidism. The body also makes enormous amounts of estrogen and progesterone during pregnancy, causing more thyroid hormones to be available to the body. The mother may also get additional benefits from the fetus, as it makes higher levels of thyroid hormones to compensate for the mother's deficiency.

Conversely, pregnancy may be very hard on the mother if she gains too much weight due to hypothyroidism. It's also common to have a very large baby when you have hypothyroidism. If a baby weighs over nine pounds at birth, it may be due to diabetes or hypothyroidism in the mother. In either case, the postpartum period can be very tough, since it's characterized by plunging levels of all hormones. Any women who experiences significant postpartum depression should have her thyroid function tested.

Libido and Sexual Function

Libido and sexual function are invariably affected by hypothyroidism. Women with inadequate thyroid function experience lack of sexual desire and satisfaction. Since thyroid hormones affect muscle and nerve activity as well as circulation, when your thyroid hormone levels are low your sexual organs aren't able to work as they should, compromising our sexual function and satisfaction. Thyroid hormone therapy has an amazing ability to reverse this situation and bring back your sex life!

WHAT'S NEXT?

Now that you fully understand the impacts of hypothyroidism on your body, we can get into the specifics of what may be affecting your thyroid function, and then how to fix it. Having an understanding of causes is important, as treatment and even deciding what tests are appropriate may vary depending on the cause of the problem. In the next chapter, we'll explore genetic, environmental, and other potential causes that could be at the root of your symptoms.

KEY POINTS

- Thyroid function affects every cell in the body and has profound effects on all of our systems and functions—physiological, mental, and emotional.

- Our appearance suffers as hair, skin, nails, teeth, weight, posture, and musculature are all negatively affected by the metabolic slowdown that occurs.

- The mind and emotions go through the same degenerative process, resulting in symptoms such as brain fog, reduced cognitive functioning, memory problems, irritability, and mood swings. More serious problems such as depression, bipolar disorder, schizophrenia, and psychosis can also result.

- Our basic body functions also undergo negative changes, affecting blood pressure, body temperature, fluid balance, digestion, elimination, heart and nerve health, breathing, liver function, mobility, and sleep.

- Hypothyroidism also affects general well-being by lowering energy levels, causing widespread pain and stiffness, and compromising immune function.

- When thyroid function is low, the reciprocity between the thyroid and the ovaries leads to various problems with reproductive function, such as menstrual problems, infertility, miscarriages, and declining libido.

CHAPTER 5

Causes of Hypothyroidism

Given the miraculous and complex functions of the thyroid gland, it's no surprise that many things can go awry and affect its ability to function properly. It's important to understand what can cause thyroid problems in order to figure out how best to test and treat them. Since women are far more likely than men to develop thyroid problems, we shouldn't be surprised that many of the causes of this malfunction arise in body parts and functions that are uniquely female—most notably our ovaries.

CHANGES IN YOUR OVARIAN FUNCTION

During perimenopause, ovarian hormone production decreases and becomes erratic. Hormone levels can veer up and down—too high one cycle and too low the next. These fluctuating levels cause a variety of menstrual changes. Your cycles can become shorter or longer, and the bleeding may be heavier or lighter. And even if your cycles remain regular, your hormone levels may still be greatly affected, leaving you with all the traditional symptoms of hormone imbalance: weight gain, brain fog, fatigue, irritability, insomnia, loss of sex drive, and on and on.

Unfortunately, it happens to all of us sooner or later. When your ovaries start to slow down in your thirties and forties, it has an overall slowing effect on your entire body, including your thyroid. This makes sense when you think back to the endocrine system and how all of its parts are so closely intertwined. Changes in any gland or the hormones it produces affect the rest of your glands. The thyroid gland has receptors for estrogen and progesterone, and it depends on the cyclic ebb and flow of these hormones throughout your menstrual cycle to function optimally. When levels of either hormone drop off, the thyroid doesn't receive the stimulation it needs to do its job properly, so thyroid hormone levels also drop. Because your thyroid is responsible for fueling all of your other glands and organs with energy, changes in ovarian function ultimately send ripples out through your entire body.

Another problem related to ovarian function occurs when you don't ovulate every cycle, which can actually happen as early as your twenties. In the cycles when you don't ovulate, you end up making only estrogen for the entire cycle, with no progesterone to balance it. Because progesterone is made by the egg sac after an egg is released at ovulation, no ovulation means no progesterone. Given that all aspects of endocrine function are connected by complex feedback loops, you can see that this will have important consequences—and it does. Estrogen has an opposing, or suppressive, effect on thyroid hormones, so when progesterone doesn't block estrogen's action for half of your cycle, chronic estrogen ends up suppressing your thyroid function. As soon as you ovulate or add supplemental progesterone for the last two weeks of the cycle, your thyroid will be able to work well again. This is one reason why perimenopause is so hard on some women. Not only are their sex hormone levels veering around wildly, but their thyroid is on the same roller coaster.

The following chart will help you visualize how important the relationship between estrogen and progesterone is.

Estrogen and progesterone levels in the menstrual cycle

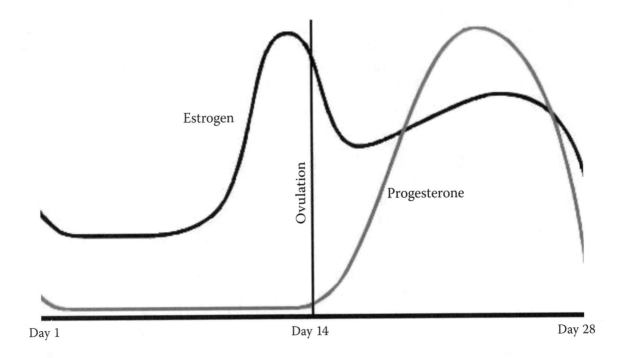

Source: Kathryn Simpson and Dale Bredesen, *The Perimenopause and Menopause Workbook* (Oakland, CA: New Harbinger Publications, 2006).

An easy solution to detecting and resolving this problem is to purchase an ovulation tester, available at any drugstore, and test whether you're ovulating in every cycle. If you're having any of the symptoms of hormone imbalance mentioned earlier, testing for ovulation could explain the cause. If you know when you fail to ovulate, you can supplement progesterone to restore the balance—if you and your doctor feel it's advisable. Suppression of your thyroid function isn't the only problem caused by irregular ovulation. Other conditions can also result from the cellular proliferation caused by estrogen when it isn't balanced by progesterone. Since this proliferation is going on everywhere in the body, not just the uterus, you can expect such things as heavy periods, mood swings, irritability, brain fog (yes, the brain is affected too), headaches, insomnia, and swollen, lumpy, sore breasts, as well as even more serious health problems, such as fibroids and endometrial, uterine, and breast cancer (Ansquer et al. 2005).

PREGNANCY

Because pregnancy is such a basic biological function for women, it may be hard to believe that it's a major risk factor for thyroid dysfunction. However, pregnancy is a huge feat for the body to accomplish, and it affects the thyroid in a number of ways. It poses a higher risk to the woman for developing both hyperthyroidism and hypothyroidism, both during and after pregnancy. Dramatic changes in levels of reproductive hormones such as estrogen and progesterone during pregnancy cause changes in thyroid hormone levels. In addition, both mother and baby require high iodine intake, and if these needs aren't met, it can result in inadequate thyroid hormone production, which can seriously affect the developing baby.

Women are also more likely to develop antibodies to their own thyroid gland during pregnancy, causing a condition known as Hashimoto's thyroiditis, or autoimmune thyroiditis ("itis" means inflammation). Immune activity is in high gear during pregnancy, and this excessive activity can cause or exacerbate an autoimmune condition in the thyroid gland. Thyroiditis is more common in the three- to six-month period after birth. It also occurs more often after miscarriages (and possibly after abortions). The incidence of miscarriage in women with thyroid antibodies is twice that of women who don't have them, so it's important to test for antibodies if you've had a miscarriage and are trying to conceive again (Marqusee, Hill, and Mandel 1997).

The classic clinical picture of pregnancy-related thyroid dysfunction is for a woman to have symptoms of hyperthyroidism during pregnancy, followed by hypothyroidism after the birth, and then a return to normal thyroid function within a year. This chain of events can cause a predisposition for the woman to develop permanent hypothyroidism later in life. Postpartum risk of developing thyroid dysfunction is also much worse in women with insulin-dependent diabetes; approximately 25 percent of these women develop thyroid problems (Alvarez-Marfany et al. 1994).

The thyroid swells during pregnancy in order to meet the higher demand for thyroid hormone required to support the baby's growth and development. A fascinating fact I came upon in an old endocrinology book was that long before pregnancy tests were available, Italian parents used to measure their daughters' necks before marriage and regularly thereafter; any increase in circumference due to a swollen thyroid was taken as a sign of pregnancy (Sajous 1903).

✔ *Julie's Story*

Julie was only thirty-five when she started to have symptoms of what she later found out was thyroid dysfunction. She'd had two children and felt fine until after the birth of her second child at thirty-four. From the time the baby was born she was exhausted. Even after she stopped nursing at six months, she still couldn't seem to regain her energy or enthusiasm for anything. She dragged through each day feeling tired and irritable. Her friends called and tried to include her in activities they used to do together before the baby was born, like going to the gym and having coffee or lunch, but Julie was too tired and depressed to do anything.

She resumed her periods after she stopped breastfeeding, but they were much lighter than they had been in the past and started every thirty to thirty-five days instead of the regular twenty-eight days she was used to.

Her relationship with her husband was also suffering, since she was depressed and irritable most of the time and couldn't summon enough energy or interest to have sex. She knew he was frustrated about the fact that she wasn't the least bit interested, but she was just too tired to make the effort. The extra thirty pounds of weight she had gained didn't help, nor did the vaginal dryness and irritation she experienced the few times they did have sex after the baby was born. She comforted herself with the thought that she was just suffering from postpartum depression. She'd heard it was a temporary condition, so she figured it would just go away on its own any day.

Unfortunately, eight months later she was still feeling the same: She had no energy or libido, and almost everything seemed to irritate her. She was having a hard time sleeping, and she was losing a huge amount of hair. She was in such a fog that she might have continued like this indefinitely, but finally her husband told her that he just couldn't take it anymore. He was sympathetic and knew the baby had taken a toll, but he didn't want to live that way and thought they should consider a separation to see if that would make her any happier. The thought of losing her husband, whom she still loved despite her frustration with him and everything else, and the thought of being on her own with two small children, shocked her into taking action. She called her doctor and scheduled an appointment.

She had no idea what to expect from the appointment, so she was incredibly relieved when, after hearing all her symptoms, her doctor told her that she was most likely suffering from hormone deficiencies or imbalances that could be diagnosed through testing and then treated. The thought that there was a solution to her misery was enough to make her feel optimistic for the first time in over a year. She immediately had the lab tests done that the doctor ordered, and then returned to his office the next week to get the results. Her doctor explained that the lab tests showed she had multiple hormone deficiencies. First and foremost, her thyroid hormone levels were significantly low, with her T4 level at rock bottom. Her TSH was very elevated, as her pituitary was working overtime trying to get her thyroid to produce hormones, and she also had high levels of thyroid antibodies. As if that weren't enough, her progesterone level showed she hadn't ovulated during that cycle, and her estrogen was very low as well.

Julie's doctor told her that the treatment for thyroid antibodies and low thyroid hormone levels was the same: taking thyroid hormones, which he prescribed in the form of Armour Thyroid, a product that contains both T3 and T4. He also prescribed bioidentical estrogen patches to raise her estrogen level to over 100 pg/ml (picograms per milliliter) and bioidentical progesterone to use the last two weeks of the month to support her menstrual cycle. Julie felt much better immediately. Her spirits lifted, she had noticeably more energy, and her hair stopped falling out. She was still tired in the afternoons and her memory wasn't as sharp as it had been before she had her baby, but her doctor explained that it could take some time and experimentation to figure out the right doses of thyroid hormones and estrogen for Julie's body.

Over the next three months, her doctor slowly increased her thyroid hormone dose. Julie also had to move up to a higher-dose estrogen patch, as her estrogen level after she started on replacement was still low. Finally, after four months, she noticed one day that she felt completely well—not one symptom was left.

PROBLEMS WITH YOUR HYPOTHALAMUS OR PITUITARY

Problems with your hypothalamus or pituitary can ultimately affect all of your other endocrine glands. Because they stimulate and regulate the activity of all the other endocrine glands, when the function of either of these important glands is affected, your thyroid function is affected too. Lots of things can cause problems with these glands. Their location right behind the nose makes them fairly easy to damage if you experience trauma to the head. This results in decreased production of regulatory hormones, which leads to inadequate stimulation of the other endocrine organs, causing low hormone levels across the board (Stratmoen 2005). This is one reason why it's so important to carefully evaluate your health history for car accidents, sports injuries, or anything else that could have damaged your hypothalamus or pituitary gland.

Other potential causes of dysfunction in the hypothalamus or pituitary are growths on one of the glands or genetic disorders. These problems can result in the gland producing insufficient or excessive amounts of various hormones.

Hypothyroidism caused by either the pituitary or the hypothalamus is known as central hypothyroidism; if caused by your pituitary, it's secondary hypothyroidism, and if caused by your hypothalamus, it's tertiary hypothyroidism. It's very important to determine where your thyroid problem originates, as this can affect how it's treated. In addition, if your pituitary or hypothalamus is causing the problem, your other endocrine glands, which are also under their control, may also be underactive. In this case, you may need to consider supplementing other hormones, including estrogen, progesterone, testosterone, and even adrenal hormones such as cortisol and DHEA.

ANTIBODIES

Antibodies are substances produced by the immune system in response to threats to your body, such as bacteria and viruses. Their job is to attack and disarm these invaders. Unfortunately, the immune system sometimes mistakes the body's own tissues for invaders. This results in the production of antibodies that attack and destroy healthy tissue by mistake. In the cases of the thyroid, it usually takes many years of this type of autoimmune activity to destroy enough of the gland to reach full-blown hypothyroidism. Because this gradual destruction of the thyroid gland tends to show up in the form of symptoms that creep up slowly and closely mimic the aging process, you may interpret them simply as signs of getting older when, in reality, your thyroid is inexorably and systematically being destroyed.

There are several different types of autoimmune thyroid diseases. Hashimoto's thyroiditis, mentioned earlier in relation to pregnancy, is the most common type of autoimmune thyroid condition. The other major type of autoimmune thyroid disease goes by the intimidating name of Graves' disease (fortunately, this is just the name of the doctor who discovered it, as opposed to any allusion to a fatal outcome). In these diseases, especially Graves' disease, there can be an initial period of hyperthyroidism as the assault of the antibodies initially causes more thyroid activity in an effort to compensate. Eventually enough of the thyroid gland is destroyed that hypothyroidism sets in. Thyroid antibodies are also more often present in women who have diabetes, rheumatoid arthritis, hepatitis, lupus, or Sjögren's syndrome.

FOREIGN INVADERS

It's thought that thyroid disease, including thyroiditis, may also be caused by viral, bacterial and fungal infections. We're constantly surrounded and invaded by microorganisms, including bacteria, viruses, and fungi. They can reside almost anywhere—our nose, throat, mouth, and intestinal tract—and we can't escape them. For the most part, we coexist with them peacefully, but when our resistance is lowered they can cause problems. Examples of bacterial infections that can be particularly harmful to your thyroid are staph, strep, salmonella, tuberculosis, and pneumonia. All sorts of viruses have been implicated in thyroid disease, including the Coxsackie virus and the viruses that cause mumps, measles, influenza, infectious mononucleosis, adenovirus, and myocarditis (De Groot, Hennemann, and Larsen 1984).

Several types of fungal infections can cause damage, the most common being candida (caused by the fungus *Candida albicans*). Overgrowth of candida is a fairly common problem in women as we age. Candida can live in the mouth, throat, genitourinary tract, and intestines, where it's considered to be a normal part of our bowel flora in its benign, yeastlike form. When it becomes infectious, it takes on a not-so-benign aggressive form.

When our hormone levels change, usually in perimenopause, the immune system can be affected due to decreased production of hormones, including the thyroid hormones and cortisol. This allows candida to get out of control and become a problem, essentially taking over the intestines.

It produces long, rootlike structures that can bore through the lining of the intestines, allowing partially digested food to escape into circulation. This causes the immune system to produce antibodies and ultimately results in autoimmune activity that further weakens the immune system. It also results in allergies to all kinds of things that hadn't caused problems before, from common foods to chemicals to pollen. It can cause other problematic conditions as well, such as leaky gut syndrome and irritable bowel syndrome.

PHYSICAL INJURY

Either indirect or direct physical injury to your thyroid gland can also cause hypothyroidism. Damage to the thyroid via indirect injury is not uncommon. Did you start to notice symptoms of hypothyroidism after a car accident that resulted in whiplash? Because the thyroid is located at the base of your neck just under the Adam's apple, if your head is jolted forward or backward in an accident or fall, it can be physically damaged. In fact, British thyroid expert Barry Durrant-Peatfield believes that 30 percent of people who have experienced whiplash will develop hypothyroidism (Durrant-Peatfield 2002). Any type of physical trauma that causes a whiplash effect can damage the thyroid.

Seat belts are one of the greatest inventions around and have saved countless lives, but studies have shown that they can also cause trauma to the neck and result in thyroid malfunction (Leckie, Buckner, and Bornemann 1992). It's important to adjust your seat belt so that it sits well under your thyroid, not over it. This is especially important for children or anyone who is shorter, causing the seatbelt to sit higher on the neck.

Of course, the thyroid can also be damaged by direct injury. Surgery on or near the thyroid gland (particularly on the parathyroid glands) often results in thyroid malfunction; for example, surgery to remove thyroid nodules, which are cysts or *adenomas* (benign overgrowths of normal tissue) on the thyroid gland. These nodules are extremely common, occurring in up to 10 percent of the adult population, and about 95 percent of them are benign (Datta, Petrelli, and Ramzy 2006; Castro and Gharib 2000). It's important to get a second opinion if your doctor recommends surgery to remove these growths, since they generally don't do any harm, whereas the surgery to remove them can easily damage your thyroid and compromise its function. If your doctor is worried about possible thyroid cancer, ask about a procedure called a needle biopsy, in which a fine needle is inserted into the thyroid gland to extract cells for evaluation. This allows diagnosis without potentially damaging your thyroid, perhaps permanently.

Here are some important questions to ask if your doctor recommends surgery to remove a growth on or near your thyroid:

- Is there any possibility that the growth could be cancerous?

- If it's not malignant, is it causing me any health problems?

- Are there any other options for treating my condition besides surgery?

🖎   What are the risks of the operation?

🖎   How much of my thyroid gland will be removed?

🖎   Will I need to take thyroid hormones after surgery?

Direct injury can occur in the form of a blow to the thyroid gland. When I go to my son's high school football games and see the kids cheering with glee when one of the players gets "clothes-lined," all I can think about is the poor boy's thyroid. Sports injuries can also affect the hypothalamus and pituitary and affect your thyroid function indirectly.

One other cause of direct injury to the thyroid gland occurs when hyperthyroidism is treated with radioactive iodine medicine. This toxic material destroys thyroid tissue and often results in hypothyroidism—an ironic but not entirely unpredictable outcome.

MEDICATIONS

Some medications damage or suppress thyroid function, including lithium, birth control pills, beta-blockers, phenytoin, theophylline, antacids that contain aluminum, sulfa drugs, antihistamines, and chemotherapy. If you must take any of these medications, work with your doctor to monitor your thyroid hormone levels carefully. Likewise, if you take supplemental estrogen, work with your doctor to make sure it's properly balanced by adequate levels of progesterone, or it will have a suppressive effect. This also applies to women who have had hysterectomies. Strangely, the prevailing medical theory is that women who have had hysterectomies don't need progesterone as they no longer have a uterus. This ignores the biological reality that whenever we have estrogen in our bodies, we must also have progesterone to balance it or the delicate and important balance of our entire endocrine system can be thrown off. When used correctly however, supplemental estrogen and progesterone are very beneficial to thyroid function, as mentioned above.

ENVIRONMENTAL TOXINS ARE EVERYWHERE

A whole new world of chemicals that are toxic to the thyroid have been created in the last fifty years. Strangely, and unfortunately, many synthetic chemicals have structures very similar to certain hormones and can fit into cellular receptors for these hormones with awesomely disruptive consequences. Many of them mimic estrogen, but some also interfere with the usage and metabolism of thyroid hormones, testosterone, and other hormones.

When your thyroid function is affected by these hormone-disrupting chemicals, it's less able to support other organs and systems, such as the immune system and liver, in doing their job of destroying poisonous substances and infectious agents. When our thyroid is working as it should, we're more able to withstand massive assaults from our environment, but when it isn't, we can't get rid of this toxic burden.

Other environmental toxins that negatively affect thyroid function include fluoride, heavy metals, and chemicals called perchlorates, which are widely found in drinking water and inhibit the production of thyroid hormones by blocking the uptake of iodine. X-rays can also be damaging. If you or your loved ones have thyroid problems, or even just suspect having them, always ask for a thyroid collar when you have any kind of X-rays—even dental.

IODINE DEFICIENCY

About 75 percent of the iodine in the your diet makes its way to your thyroid gland. It's critical in manufacturing both T3 and T4, so iodine deficiency can result in hypothyroidism. Long-term iodine deficiency can result in an enlarged thyroid gland, known as a goiter, which develops when the thyroid gland gets bigger in an attempt to increase the output of thyroid hormones. Goiters often get large enough to be seen at the base of the neck. In the extreme, severe iodine deficiency in children results in mental retardation, a condition rare in developed countries like the United States.

Since iodine has been added to the U.S. food supply—first to bread and milk and then switched to table salt—most people believe that iodine deficiency isn't an issue here. Unfortunately, the most recent National Health and Nutrition Examination Survey, from 1994, showed that the average U.S. daily intake of iodine has fallen by more than 50 percent in the past twenty years—from 320 mcg (micrograms) to 145 mcg. The study showed that 14.9 percent of adult women were deficient in iodine, a 4.5-fold increase over the rate in 1974 (Hollowell et al. 1998).

This deficiency may due to the fact that many people now restrict their salt intake because of the connection between salt and hypertension. Also, in years past we got plenty of additional iodine from vegetables grown in iodine-rich soil, but intensive farming practices have robbed our soil of iodine and other minerals, resulting in produce that's low in iodine and many other important minerals.

Finally, even if you use iodized salt, to get the recommended daily allowance (RDA) for iodine, 150 mcg for adults, you'd need to use a little more than 1/2 teaspoon of iodized salt daily—something you may not be willing to do because of other health issues. Another concern is that the chloride in salt competes with iodine for absorption, so we may not be able to readily absorb all of the iodine present in iodized salt. Plus, recent research suggests that even this RDA may be too low to produce sufficient thyroid hormones (Abraham, Flechas, and Hakala 2002).

Iodine deficiency has ramifications beyond your thyroid, too. Because iodine is utilized by every hormone receptor in the body, inadequate iodine intake can result in widespread hormonal imbalances, causing problems such as ovarian cysts, goiter, and thyroid adenomas. If you don't use much salt, it's best to take supplemental iodine. Another good source of iodine is seafood and seaweeds, such as nori and kelp.

GENETICS

Genetic factors can play a role in hypothyroidism. An inherited thyroid deficiency is often the cause of low thyroid function. In addition, there's a possibility that impaired thyroid function in a parent—due to any cause—may be passed along to his or her children. So you may have increased risk of thyroid dysfunction if either of your parents was subject to any of the other causes of hypothyroidism. Notably, these include a drinking problem, excessive exposure to X-rays, chemotherapy, or physical damage.

Familial thyroid dysfunction can manifest in very different conditions and symptoms in different family members. For instance, you might have hypothyroidism or Hashimoto's disease, and your child may have Graves' disease. If you or any other blood relatives have a thyroid condition, be on the lookout for signs and symptoms of any type of thyroid dysfunction in you and your children. The following exercise will help you determine whether your family history gives cause for concern.

EXERCISE: Family Health History

All of the following symptoms can be indicative of hypothyroidism. In the space provided, note whether each symptom has affected any of your family members. You can code them as follows: M = mother, F = father, B = brother, S = sister, GF = grandfather, GM = grandmother, A = aunt, U = uncle.

_____ Adrenal dysfunction

_____ Alcoholism

_____ Allergies

_____ Alzheimer's disease

_____ Anemia

_____ Anxiety

_____ Arthritis

_____ Asthma

_____ Attention-deficit/hyperactivity disorder (ADHD)

_____ Autoimmune disease

_____ Back pain

_____ Bipolar disorder

_____ Bladder problems

_____ Breathing difficulties

_____ Cancer

_____ Carpal tunnel syndrome

_____ Chemical dependency

_____ Chronic constipation or diarrhea

_____ Chronic fatigue

_____ Chronic shortness of breath

_____ Defective nails

_____ Dementia

_____ Depression

_____ Diabetes

_____ Difficult menopause

_____ Difficulty concentrating

_____ Difficulty swallowing

_____ Early hair graying	_____ Liver disorders
_____ Easy bleeding or bruising	_____ Memory loss
_____ Eating disorder	_____ Menstrual cycle disorders
_____ Elevated cholesterol or triglycerides	_____ Mental illness
_____ Emphysema	_____ Neurological disorders
_____ Epilepsy or seizures	_____ Osteoporosis
_____ Eye and vision problems	_____ Panic attacks
_____ Fibrocystic breasts	_____ Pneumonia
_____ Fibroids	_____ Protuberant eyes
_____ Fibromyalgia	_____ Recurrent infections
_____ Gallbladder disease	_____ Respiratory disorders
_____ Goiter	_____ Restless legs syndrome
_____ Gout	_____ Schizophrenia
_____ Headaches or migraines	_____ Severe hair loss
_____ Hearing problems	_____ Sinus problems
_____ Heart attack	_____ Skin problems
_____ Heart disease	_____ Stomach or gastrointestinal disorders
_____ Heartburn or acid reflux	_____ Stunted growth
_____ Hemorrhoids	_____ Thin hair
_____ High blood pressure	_____ Thyroid dysfunction
_____ Hypoglycemia	_____ Tobacco smoker
_____ Inflammatory bowel disease	_____ Tuberculosis
_____ Insomnia	_____ Unexplained weight loss
_____ Jaundice	_____ Vertigo, dizziness, or light-headedness
_____ Joint pain or stiffness	_____ Vocal problems
_____ Leg pain	_____ Weight gain or obesity

Take a copy of this completed Family Health History with you when you meet with your doctor so he or she will have a thorough understanding of possible inherited predisposition for thyroid dysfunction. If you noted multiple symptoms for any relatives, you can better assess whether that person has a thyroid problem by having them complete the Hypothyroidism Symptom Evaluation in chapter 3.

CONVERSION PROBLEMS

As you may recall from chapter 1, T4 has low biologic activity and the body converts a great deal of it into the more active T3. This conversion process takes place in many organs, including the brain, liver, and kidneys, via the enzyme iodothyronine 5'-deiodinase. This process can be hampered by a fairly large number of problems, including inflammation, fasting, malnutrition (including that due to digestive problems), heavy metal toxicity, growth hormone deficiency, cigarette smoking, kidney or liver dysfunction, trauma, chronic illness, vitamin and mineral deficiencies, chemotherapy, elevated levels of cortisol or sex-hormone-binding globulin, and excess estrogen (from birth control pills or estrogen replacement not balanced by progesterone).

Since so many things can affect this conversion process, many of which are caused by inadequate levels of thyroid hormone to begin with, it's important to measure levels of T3 when you have your thyroid function tested. This can help determine whether you have a conversion problem, in which case it's probably best to supplement with a product that contains both T3 and T4.

Another conversion problem is that T4 can be converted to reverse T3 (rT3) instead of the active T3. (Reverse T3 is stereoisomer of T3, meaning it has the same chemical makeup as T3 but an opposite rotation, so it's a mirror image of T3.) Conversion of T4 to rT3 can be caused by many of the same things that block conversion of T4 to T3. Because the shape of reverse T3 is different than regular T3, it doesn't have the same biological activity; however, it can still bind to T3 receptors and prevent them from binding T3. As a result, excess rT3 effectively blocks the body's ability to use the T3 it does make, so even if your T3 levels are high, you'll still have impaired thyroid function. Chapter 6 will provide full details on testing for these conversion disorders, and chapter 7 will discuss their treatment.

THYROID HORMONE RESISTANCE

T3 has to enter your cells via its receptors in order to have an effect on your body. As discussed above, rT3 can block these receptors. In addition, sometimes unoccupied receptors fail to bind T3. The reasons for this are unknown (though it is possibly genetic), but the end result is hypothyroidism. This is impossible to easily diagnose, as it would require measuring thyroid levels in the cells, which isn't currently possible. The one indicator to look for in lab tests is high T3 and T4 levels combined with a normal TSH level, showing that thyroid hormones aren't able to enter the cells and are building up in the bloodstream.

The only treatment for this condition is higher than normal doses of supplemental thyroid hormones to offset the resistance of the cells (Lowe 2000). Doctors who test and treat this condition find that when these patients take higher doses of hormones, they don't show signs of hyperthyroidism, even though their lab tests indicate it. In fact, this is one of the ways they determine whether the diagnosis is correct. This isn't currently a commonly accepted practice, so you'd need to work with a trained thyroid practitioner to investigate and treat this condition.

Another receptor problem occurs when your receptors become desensitized due to long-term hypothyroidism. This can also be caused or exacerbated by low cortisol levels. So it's important to measure levels of thyroid hormones and cortisol together.

ADRENAL COMPLICATIONS

Cortisol, produced by the adrenal glands, is necessary for converting T4 to T3. It also ensures thyroid receptor function, as the receptors can become defunct or even disappear in the absence of good adrenal function. So without enough cortisol, you can't use the thyroid hormones you do make very well. As a result, most women with long-term or severe hypothyroidism should be evaluated for adrenal insufficiency, which should be treated at the same time as hypothyroidism. See chapter 9 for a full discussion of the relationship between adrenal function and thyroid function.

WHAT'S NEXT?

Now that you have a good sense of how well your thyroid is functioning, an understanding of your symptoms, and some ideas about possible causes, it's time to do something about it. If you haven't already had your thyroid function tested, that's the next step, as the information from lab tests is important for designing an effective treatment plan. The next chapter will provide full details on all of the necessary tests and how to interpret them. It will also discuss some of the shortcomings inherent in hormone testing.

KEY POINTS

❦ Decreasing ovarian hormone production, as well as erratic ovarian function, has an overall slowing effect on the entire body, including the thyroid.

❦ Hypothyroidism can also be caused by pregnancy, malfunction of the pituitary or hypothalamus, thyroid antibodies, infections, direct or indirect injury to the thyroid gland, medications, environmental toxins, iodine deficiency, genetic predisposition, conversion problems, resistance to thyroid hormones at the cell receptor level, and adrenal complications.

❦ It's important to look at your family history in order to understand fully your risk for potentially developing thyroid disease. An inherited thyroid deficiency is often the cause of low thyroid function. You may have increased risk of thyroid dysfunction if either of your parents had hypothyroidism caused by things such as a drinking problem, excessive exposure to X-rays, chemotherapy, or physical damage.

❦ Inherited thyroid dysfunction can cause different problems in different family members. It may show up as hypothyroidism, Hashimoto's disease, or even Graves' disease. If you or any other family members have a thyroid problem, be on the lookout for signs and symptoms in other family members.

CHAPTER 6

Thyroid Testing Made Simple

Have you seen your doctor and been told that your thyroid is functioning just fine and that the myriad of symptoms that have kept you on a merry-go-round of doctor visits, blood tests, ultrasounds, and even CAT scans and MRIs are caused by confusing-sounding things like IBS, PMS, MS, ADHD, or PVD? I heard almost every one of these acronyms bandied about by my doctors, and all the while I got no closer to solving my health problems. And yet all of these confusing-sounding conditions are actually related to low thyroid function. The thing is, once you're labeled with one of these intimidating acronyms, the investigation concludes and, most likely, you're given a prescription (or multiple prescriptions) for drugs to help manage the symptoms. Thyroid health or other underlying causes are seldom considered.

One of the main problems in detecting thyroid disorders is that thyroid testing has become a confusing tangle of conflicting information instead of the useful tool it should be. Rather than helping you get to the bottom of what's going on and clarifying the path to correct any problems you may have, it may feel like a seemingly incomprehensible and insurmountable hurdle in your quest for thyroid health. And yet blood tests and other laboratory tests are a crucial tool for getting to the bottom of the situation and developing an effective treatment plan.

In this chapter, I'll clear up some of the confusion by describing the various laboratory tests and their results in detail. But first, let's take a look at some of the issues that affect the usefulness of lab tests.

CUTTING THROUGH THE CONFUSION AROUND THYROID TESTING

If the evaluations and simple self-tests in chapter 3 indicated you may have a thyroid problem, the next step is to work with a doctor to test your thyroid function and decide on the best treatment plan. As mentioned, the lab tests involved can seem very confusing and difficult to interpret. To optimize your chances for success and help you arrive at a solution more quickly, it's important to choose the right doctor, and to understand some of the inherent limitations and difficulties of the lab tests.

Choosing the Right Doctor

The first inadvertent mistake many of us make when we start the process of evaluating our thyroid health is underestimating the importance of choosing the right doctor to guide us through this maze. We blithely assume any old doctor will do, that our internist or ob-gyn will serendipitously understand the ins and outs of our thyroid. But in reality, very few doctors are trained in thyroid testing and treatment. It can be a simple matter to figure out what's wrong and devise an appropriate treatment plan—*if* your doctor has studied and practiced thyroid hormone therapy for years. However, doctors who haven't can't possibly untangle the mass of new research data that has emerged regarding thyroid health in the last decade alone. For many doctors, it simply isn't practical or possible to spend hours at the end of a ten- to twelve-hour workday reading medical journals. And even if they did, the subtleties of testing and treating thyroid dysfunction are only apparent after a lot of practice. Do you really want to be the one your doctor is practicing on?

The better course is to do your homework up front and find a doctor who has been treating thyroid problems and other hormone issues for years. A seasoned doctor will understand the importance of comprehensive thyroid evaluation and testing, rather than settling for just a TSH test and maybe a T4 test. You won't have to fight for tests and treatment at every turn. Doctors are understandably uncomfortable using treatments they aren't familiar with, so those who don't specialize in thyroid treatment generally fall back on treatments they are familiar with, such as using antidepressant drugs to muffle your symptoms.

Understanding Test Results, and Their Limitations

There are many reasons why thyroid testing can lead doctors and their patients astray. The first is that the right tests to get to the root of the problem often aren't done. And even if they are, there is no absolute "right" or "wrong" level for everyone. Each of us has a unique biological makeup; a hormone level that is fine for one woman may be far too low for another. So test results don't tell the whole story.

Another big problem is that the reference ranges used by large testing labs and relied upon by many doctors to determine whether your levels are "normal" are often outdated and incorrect.

Unfortunately, doctors who don't specialize in thyroid treatment don't understand this, so they tend to overlook many cases of hypothyroidism.

And finally, as any doctor will tell you, a blood test is only a snapshot of what's going on at the time samples are taken, whether of blood, urine, or saliva. Your test may show varying levels of different hormones depending on what time of day you take the test, what you've had to eat or drink, how much sleep you've had, and even how hot it is on the day samples are taken.

In fact, one research study showed that TSH levels go down significantly later in the day, by an average of about 26 percent, compared to results in the morning after fasting. This may not seem all that important, but it actually resulted in 6 percent of the participants being reclassified from a diagnosis of hypothyroidism to "normal" (Scobbo et al. 2004). This means that if you get tested later in the day while not fasting, your TSH level will be lower, indicating a more robust thyroid function than you actually may have. (Remember, TSH is thyroid-stimulating hormone, so lower levels mean your body has more thyroid hormones.)

It isn't realistic for you to control all of the factors that could affect your results (such as the outside temperature the day you go in for your test!), but you should try to control as many variables as you can. One important way to do this is to always have blood samples taken first thing in the morning while fasting.

Most doctors who specialize in thyroid treatment agree that test results shouldn't be the only deciding factor in evaluating thyroid function. They're an important tool, but they should be used to validate clinical impressions, not as the sole basis for a diagnosis. So, keeping all of these caveats in mind, let's take a look at the various laboratory tests that can be helpful in assessing thyroid function.

LABORATORY TESTS FOR THYROID FUNCTION

The great majority of doctors who test thyroid levels test only TSH. This is indeed an important hormone to test, as high levels indicate that your pituitary gland is sensing a lack of adequate thyroid hormones in your body, so it's trying to stimulate your thyroid to make more. However, if the problem isn't with your thyroid but actually originates in your hypothalamus, pituitary, thyroid hormone receptors, or elsewhere, this test won't detect the problem. Recent research suggests that as many as one in five people worldwide have a pituitary disease or disorder, and most of them don't even know it (Pituitary Network Organization 2007). And, if your pituitary isn't working right, neither will your thyroid.

Many doctors will also test levels of T4, but usually only total levels, not free levels. The latter is important, as it measures the amount of T4 not bound up by proteins and therefore available to your cells. Doctors who don't specialize in the treatment of thyroid disorders often don't realize this. In addition, it's also necessary to test levels of free T3 and, in many cases, levels of thyroid antibodies and reverse T3. Once you understand the importance of each of these tests, it will be easier for you to discuss these issues with potential doctors and determine whether they have the right background and knowledge to evaluate your thyroid function effectively.

Thyroid-Stimulating Hormone (TSH) Test

The TSH test is a simple blood test. As discussed above, TSH levels go up when the body isn't making enough T3 and T4 thyroid hormones.

The relationship between TSH, T4, and T3

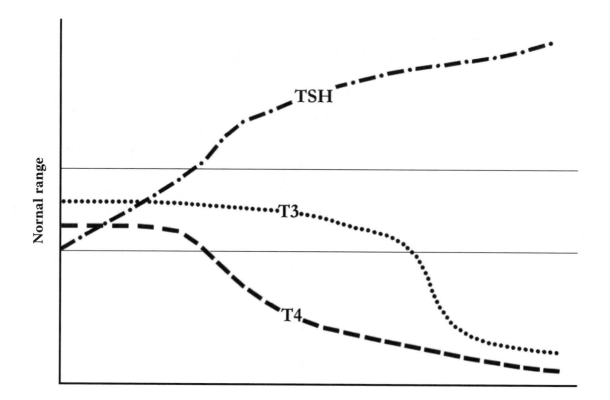

The problem with relying on TSH levels as the final word on how your thyroid is functioning is that TSH production can be affected by many factors other than levels of T3 and T4. First of all, if your thyroid dysfunction is caused by a malfunction of your pituitary or hypothalamus, these glands won't respond normally to a thyroid hormone deficiency, with the end result that your pituitary won't produce TSH when it's needed. So your TSH levels can look great even when you're deficient in thyroid hormones.

Another problem with using only TSH levels to assess your thyroid function is that exposure to certain chemicals can affect its production. Let's start with the premise that everything in the body is attached, related, regulated, or otherwise affected by everything else. This is so pervasive that it's probable we'll never understand all the connections. We do know, however, that among the many factors affecting the thyroid receptors are a group of proteins called G1 proteins. Unfortunately, environmental exposure to certain chemicals can make these proteins go haywire and cause the body to reduce TSH production even if thyroid hormone levels are too low.

The most common of these chemicals is fluoride, which is added to much of our water supply (Li 2003). Other chemicals that affect these proteins are aluminum, silica, and beryllium. It's wise to try to limit your exposure to these chemicals, but it can be difficult, as they're becoming ever more widespread in our environment. If your tap water is fluoridated, it's best to filter your drinking water or drink bottled water. Be aware that not all water filters remove fluoride, so make sure you purchase one that does. Many toothpastes also contain fluoride, and well-meaning pediatricians often recommend fluoride supplements for children, for protection against tooth decay.

As mentioned earlier, another problem with TSH testing is that many of the large labs use outdated reference ranges. Most doctors who don't specialize in hormones will see that the patient is within the "normal" range and therefore miss many potential cases of hypothyroidism. This is one reason why so many people suffering from hypothyroidism are told that their overwhelming symptoms are all in their mind.

Most experts and doctors who treat thyroid disease now believe that these old reference ranges are inaccurate. Research has shown that the reference populations (the group of people tested to decide what the normal ranges were) contained many people who had varying degrees of thyroid dysfunction, which increased the mean TSH levels for the whole group (Wartofsky and Dickey 2005). This resulted in "normal" ranges that are much higher than they should be for TSH and lower than they should be for T3 and T4.

Recent guidelines from the National Academy of Clinical Biochemistry indicate that more than 95 percent of normal individuals have TSH levels lower than 2.5 mU/l (milliunits per liter; Wartofsky and Dickey 2005). They believe that the remaining 5 percent, who have higher levels, should be excluded from the pool used to establish the reference ranges, as Hashimoto's thyroiditis or some other illness may be responsible for their higher TSH levels. Supporting this position is the fact that African-Americans, who have a very low incidence of Hashimoto's thyroiditis, have a mean TSH level of 1.18 mU/l, which is thought to be closer to the true normal mean (Wartofsky and Dickey 2005). Many labs still use a "normal" reference range of 0.3 to 5.0 mU/l (or even 6.0 mU/l). This means that people who fall between 2.5 and 6.0 mU/l are being incorrectly told their level is fine, when in reality they're probably suffering from hypothyroidism.

Free T3 and T4 Tests

In the blood, almost all T3 (99.5 percent) is bound to carrier proteins. The remaining 0.5 percent of free, unbound T3 is believed to be responsible for the hormone's biological action. Levels of carrier proteins change for various reasons, including taking birth control pills or estrogen therapy, which increase amounts of these proteins. As a result, *total* T3 levels change, but *free* T3 levels remain constant. This is one reason why free T3 is a better indication of your thyroid status than total T3.

Even if you have your free T3 level tested, you must realize that free T3 test results have some of the same problems as TSH test results, especially the "what is normal" conundrum. There is a big disparity between different sources on "normal" ranges for free T3. The following "normal" reference ranges (expressed in picograms per deciliter) illustrate how serious this problem is:

- National Academy of Clinical Biochemistry: 200–500 pg/dl

- Diagnostic Automation: 140–420 pg/dl

- Quest Diagnostic Lab and LabCorp: 230–420 pg/dl

- Siemens Medical Solutions: 150–410 pg/dl

All of these sources suggest that if you fall within the range, your T3 levels are normal. That doesn't tell the whole story, however. First, if your doctor uses Diagnostic Automation's range and your result is 140 pg/dl, you would be deemed normal, whereas you would need a level of 230 to be normal according to some of the largest testing labs, such as Quest Diagnostics and LabCorp. Second, you can be "normal" with a free T3 of 231 and still feel awful if your individual requirement for T3 is higher. Since the range for normal goes up to 500 in some cases, maybe that's the level you need to be normal. The same issues affect T4 tests.

Reverse T3 Test

Your thyroid produces more T4 than any other thyroid hormone. Most of it is converted into T3, but some is converted into reverse T3 (rT3) as a way to help clear T4 from the body. If you're deficient in vitamins, minerals, and fatty acids, or if you have high levels of toxic metals such as mercury and cadmium, your body may have a harder time converting T4 to T3 and instead convert a greater amount of T4 to rT3.

This is fine in times of starvation, when the body is valiantly trying to reduce its metabolic rate in order to get by until food is plentiful again. In such cases, making a lot of rT3 is lifesaving, but as this is not the case for most of us, it's extremely detrimental because we end up with too low a metabolic rate to feel good and remain healthy. Unfortunately, illness, high cortisol production due to stress, and excessive dieting (which the body reads as famine) all have the same effect of inhibiting the conversion of T4 to T3 and increasing the conversion of T4 to rT3. As mentioned in chapter 5, rT3 doesn't have biological activity, but it does bind with T3 receptors and thereby block the action of T3. So it's advisable to measure rT3 levels as well as free T3 levels to get a complete picture. Measuring rT3 levels is an easy blood test.

Thyroid Antibody Tests

Simple blood tests are available to test to see if your immune system is producing antibodies that may be attacking your thyroid as if it were a foreign invader, which can impair its function. Several different types of thyroid antibodies should be measured if you have symptoms of thyroid dysfunction: thyroglobulin antibodies (TgAb), and thyroid peroxidase antibodies (TPOAb), are implicated in hypothyroidism. For hyperthyroidism, on the other hand, it's important to also test for TSH receptor antibodies (TRAb), which are implicated in Graves' disease.

There is some controversy surrounding thyroid antibodies, as a small percentage of people who have them don't develop symptoms of thyroid dysfunction. Because of this, some doctors don't believe in testing for them. However, the great majority of women with antibodies do experience symptoms eventually. If you test positive for thyroid antibodies, this fact should definitely be taken into consideration when deciding if treatment is necessary.

Further confounding the issue are recent studies showing that blood tests sometimes fail to detect autoimmune hypothyroidism. One Swedish study looked at people with symptoms of hypothyroidism but "normal" blood tests for TSH, thyroid hormones, and thyroid antibodies. Small samples of thyroid tissue (taken with a needle) showed evidence of autoimmune thyroid disease in the tissues of many of the subjects (Wikland 2008a, 2008b; Sandberg 2008). This suggests that symptoms may be a more accurate indicator of thyroid dysfunction than lab tests in some cases of hypothyroidism.

Thyroid hormone therapy is helpful in reducing autoimmune antibody activity, as it lowers the need for the thyroid to make thyroid hormones. The decrease in autoimmune activity reduces inflammation in the thyroid gland. Plus, the supplemental thyroid hormones will help stimulate a higher rate of metabolic activity.

Thyroxine-Binding Globulin (TBG) Test

A TBG test is a blood test that measures the level of thyroxine-binding globulin (TBG), a protein manufactured in the liver. TBG binds to T3 and T4 and helps transport them throughout your body and releases them wherever they're needed to regulate body functions. And when T3 and T4 are bound to TBG, the kidneys don't remove them from the blood,

Pregnancy, certain diseases such as viral hepatitis, and several drugs, including steroids, affect TBG levels. Abnormal TBG levels cause total T4 and T3 levels to be abnormal but don't affect levels of free T3 and T4. Therefore, this test usually isn't necessary if levels of free T3 and free T4 are tested.

Thyrotropin-Releasing Hormone (TRH) Test

The TRH test is done to detect secondary or tertiary hypothyroidism, caused by damage to the pituitary or hypothalamus, respectively. TRH is made in your hypothalamus and is responsible for directing the production and secretion of TSH by your pituitary. If your hypothalamus doesn't make enough TRH, your body won't make enough thyroid hormones. If you have obvious thyroid symptoms but normal TSH test results, a TRH test can detect the root of the problem.

In this test, a baseline TSH blood test will be done first. Then you'll be given an injection of TRH to stimulate your pituitary to release more TSH, after which your levels of TSH will be measured at several subsequent points. This test gives an indication of how your thyroid performs when stimulated. If the function of your hypothalamus or pituitary is compromised, you may have a delayed, blunted, or even absent response to the administration of TRH.

Iodine Loading Test

The iodine loading test is a twenty-four-hour urine test used to detect whether iodine deficiency may be causing or exacerbating thyroid dysfunction. It's done at home using a kit that's mailed to you or given to you by your doctor. First, you take a 50 mg (milligram) iodine pill, then you collect all of your urine over the next twenty-four hours. This urine sample will be tested at a lab for levels of iodine. If you have enough iodine for your body's needs, most of the ingested iodine will be excreted in your urine over the twenty-four-hour period. If you're deficient in iodine, you'll retain a greater percentage of the supplemental iodine. The test is a good indicator of whether you need more iodine to get the most out of your thyroid function.

Always Check Your Estrogen and Progesterone Levels First!

As discussed in chapter 5, when estrogen isn't balanced by enough progesterone, it suppresses your thyroid function. Therefore, a deficiency of progesterone can be the root cause of hypothyroidism. Before you start on thyroid hormone therapy, you should always have your levels of estrogen and progesterone tested to see if this imbalance may be causing your symptoms. If it is, work with your doctor to come up with an appropriate program for supplementing progesterone in the last two weeks of your cycle. And lastly, you should also test levels of testosterone and follicle-stimulating hormone (FSH) as well to get a complete picture of your ovarian hormone status.

WHAT'S NEXT?

Time to get tested. If your doctor is experienced with thyroid disorders and the testing involved, great! If not, the Resources section includes information on how to find a doctor who does have the necessary experience. Take your completed symptom evaluation from chapter 3 to your appointment to give your doctor a complete picture of how your thyroid is functioning. If the Family Health History in chapter 5 indicated that any of your blood relatives may have thyroid problems, take that evaluation with you as well. Lab tests are important, but your symptoms and risk factors are just as important. If you have significant symptoms of thyroid dysfunction, such as goiter, bipolar disorder, fertility problems, or a family history of thyroid problems, many doctors who specialize in thyroid treatment will agree to a trial course of thyroid hormone therapy even if your lab test results are "normal."

Remember, it's always important to evaluate your adrenal function when you evaluate your thyroid function—initially as well as periodically during thyroid treatment (see chapter 9 for more on this). Because of the interrelationships between all of the endocrine glands and their hormones, it would be a good idea to test levels of other key hormones as well, such as estrogen, progesterone, and testosterone. A knowledgeable doctor should be able to assess which tests are needed based on your symptoms.

Once you've found a good doctor to work with and have had the needed lab tests, you're in the home stretch. All that remains is to put together an appropriate treatment plan and monitor the results—the topic of the next chapter.

KEY POINTS

ᕮ Thyroid testing is an important part of a complete thyroid evaluation, but it has several fairly significant drawbacks. Thyroid tests don't detect many types of thyroid dysfunction that might be resolved by thyroid hormone therapy. Outdated reference ranges are still in widespread use, causing a huge amount of misdiagnosis and confusion. Plus, there are no absolute "right" or "wrong" levels; every woman has a unique biological makeup. And finally, a blood test is only a snapshot of what's going on at the exact moment you have your blood drawn and may not give a complete picture.

ᕮ Thyroid tests are an important tool, but a thorough assessment of symptoms and risk factors is also essential for an accurate diagnosis.

ᕮ The following tests are necessary for a complete understanding of your thyroid health: TSH, free T3, free T4, reverse T3, and thyroid antibodies (TgAb and TPOAb or, for hyperthyroidism, TRAb).

ᕮ Always take a complete list of your symptoms, health history, and family health history with you to appointments so you can share this information with your doctor as part of a thorough evaluation of your thyroid function.

CHAPTER 7

Treatment Options for Hypothyroidism

If the information and exercises you've read so far suggest you may have hypothyroidism, it's important that you evaluate what therapy options are available and which might be the best for you personally. At this point, you may be grinding your teeth and thinking, "Just tell me what to take and be done with it!" But it's in your best interests to educate yourself about the different thyroid products available to treat hypothyroidism and what effect they have. If, after finally being accurately diagnosed, you end up with the wrong therapy, the result can be less than optimal improvement, or even no improvement at all.

The right thyroid hormone therapy will speed up your heart rate, bringing blood to all of your tissues and organs, stimulating assimilation of nutrients as well as elimination, clearing up skin and hair problems, and affecting your appearance, health, and well-being. With the right medication, you'll start to feel better almost immediately. In fact, you may experience a drastic reduction of many of your symptoms within the first month.

THE GREAT THYROID THERAPY DEBATE (T3 VS. T4)

To most effectively resolve all of your symptoms, it's important to find the right medicine, as well as the best daily dosage and dosing schedule. If you go to a doctor experienced in thyroid therapy, he or she will understand and be able to explain the options and recommend the one that best suits your condition. If you aren't able to see such a doctor due to finances, insurance requirements, or other issues, you're likely to end up being prescribed a drug consisting of T4 only, such as Synthroid, Levothroid, and Levoxyl (all brand names for levothyroxine), which have been some of the best-selling drugs in the United States for decades.

Problems with T4-Only Treatment

Unfortunately, T4 alone isn't enough to resolve symptoms for many women. Some women, particularly those with robust ovarian function (in other words, not perimenopausal or menopausal women) will do well on T4 alone, but many women require T3 supplementation as well. Recent research has shown that many women have a hard time converting T4 to T3 because of factors such as stress, diet, and illness (De Groot 1999). Another complication is that certain enzymes are necessary for the conversion of T4 into T3. The sympathetic nervous system affects the ability of these enzymes to accomplish this conversion. Because sympathetic nervous system activity is reduced in obese people, a T4-only drug may also not be the best solution for you if you're overweight (Spraul et al. 1993).

Another limitation of T4-only products is that they won't address problems due to excessive conversion of T4 to reverse T3. In this situation, adding only T4 can actually exacerbate the problem and cause more production of reverse T3, further blocking the body's ability to use the T3 it does have. Clinical studies suggest that many people have better results with thyroid hormone therapy that includes T3 (Bunevicius et al. 1999).

Barry Durrant-Peatfield, a remarkable doctor in the United Kingdom who has been treating thyroid disorders for many decades, has seen treatment fads come and go. In his book *The Great Thyroid Scandal and How to Survive It* (2002), he states that in his long clinical experience, T4 therapy is generally only effective in early, mild cases of hypothyroidism, whereas in more serious cases it isn't nearly as beneficial as a product that also contains T3. This is because T4 isn't as effective in treating complications such as low adrenal function, hormone receptor resistance, and conversion problems. He goes on to say that while using T4-only therapy, "the patient may feel an initial benefit, but within days or weeks this may wear off; or the person may soon start to become aware of tremors and palpitations. The blood test may well show the presence of too much thyroid in the blood—since it is not being used—and the dose will be reduced. This makes the side effects better but the exhaustion and fluid retention and all the other symptoms will still be there, poorly relieved, if at all. This is the situation that I found in about 70 percent of the patients [already on treatment] I saw for the first time" (Durrant-Peatfield 2002, 114). If you can't convert T4 to T3 or your receptors aren't letting thyroid hormones into your cells, it makes sense that levels of T4 might build up when you supplement it, as it effectively has nowhere to go.

Thierry Hertoghe, MD, a fourth-generation Belgian endocrine physician, has also worked with thyroid hormone therapy for decades. (His great-grandfather was one of the first endocrinologists to study thyroid function.) Dr. Hertoghe states that combination drugs may work better than a drug that contains only T4, as they enhance conversion of T4 to T3, are better absorbed, and have better potency and stability. In addition, they are more effective at accomplishing the following (Hertoghe 2006):

- Lowering total cholesterol
- Normalizing the Achilles tendon reflex
- Preventing the formation of goiters

🖎 Controlling symptoms in some clinical studies

🖎 Raising levels of T3 for better metabolic stimulation of the heart, lung, spleen, muscles, ovaries, and adrenals

Other practitioners disagree with Drs. Durrant-Peatfield and Hertoghe, but given their long-term experience with thyroid treatment, you may want to keep this advice in mind if you don't experience total resolution of your symptoms with a T4-only medication.

Your free T3 level is also a key factor in whether you need to use a T4-only drug or a T3/T4 combination drug. Another consideration is your response to thyroid therapy. If your free T3 level is robust (optimally above 350 pg/dl) and you don't have elevated reverse T3, your doctor may want you to try T4-only therapy first. If this doesn't completely resolve your symptoms, then it's a good idea to try a T3/T4 combination drug to see if you get better results—even if your T3 level is robust and you don't have elevated reverse T3.

A Historical Perspective

In my research on hormone health, I came across some information in medical books from the early 1900s that put the situation in a unique historical perspective. In 1937, it was reported that "synthetic thyroxine [T4], which has recently been introduced, appears to possess no advantages over the dried gland preparations—in fact, the majority of clinicians would probably agree that it is of distinctly less value" (Gardiner-Hill 1937, 132). Another endocrine specialist added "that 'crude' desiccated thyroid has come back to replace its more refined descendant [T4]. This cycle has been repeated a number of times in the history of endocrinology, and the recalling of it should save us from the possible error of discarding a tried-and-true endocrine product in favor of a more highly purified fraction from which essential elements may have been discarded" (Harrower 1939, 19). It looks like we still haven't learned our lesson!

Why Such Controversy over Prescribing T3 as Well as T4?

For many doctors, prescribing a T4-only drug is a simple legal issue related to standard-of-care. The term "standard of care" means practicing medicine as "the average, prudent provider in a given community would practice. It is how similarly qualified practitioners would have managed the patient's care under the same or similar circumstances" (MedicineNet 2008). These days, drug companies drive what becomes the standard of care by obtaining FDA approval for their drugs and then publicizing and marketing these therapies, resulting in widespread use. This makes it prudent for doctors to stick with these therapies in order to lessen their medical malpractice risk, an important consideration for them, given that malpractice insurance has become so expensive, and the risk of being sued so high.

This is a very understandable concern, so to ensure that you have access to the best possible hormone therapy (which may not be the standard-of-care T4-only drugs), you need to do your part and agree to partner with your doctor in taking responsibility for your treatment. In order to try a T3/T4 drug, you may have to sign a waiver or informed consent form stating that you understand that you're trying a non-standard-of-care therapy and that you've been notified of this.

Another problem is that there's a lot of confusion in the medical community involving one of the most popular T3/T4 combination drugs, Armour Thyroid. For many years, pharmaceutical sales representatives for the companies that make synthetic thyroid medications have been telling doctors that their products are superior to desiccated thyroid products such as Armour, which are made from porcine thyroid glands. They claim that these products are unstable, and because these sales representatives are the primary source of information about drugs for most doctors, many doctors have repeated these concerns to their patients, believing them to be true. This rumor continues to spread, despite the fact that the quality record of Armour Thyroid is far better than that of T4-only drugs. Meanwhile, despite this rumor, desiccated thyroid products have become increasingly popular because of women spreading the word about their experiences.

THYROID PRODUCTS ON THE MARKET

There are three categories of supplemental thyroid hormones available: T4-only products, available in many brand and generic versions, T3/T4 combination products, and T3-only drugs, which can be used alone or with a T4 drug.

T4-Only Products

T4 drugs, such as Synthroid, Levothroid, and Levoxyl, are generally dosed in micrograms, although sometimes they're prescribed in milligrams. To convert milligrams to micrograms, move the decimal point three places to the right. For example, 0.15 mg equals 150 mcg. Most doctors recommend doses of 1 mcg per pound of body weight. So if you weigh 125 pounds, you might ultimately be prescribed 125 mcg of T4. As with all thyroid drugs, your doctor will probably start you at a lower dose and raise it slowly to find your optimal dose. Many doctors start as low as 25 to 50 mcg and raise the dose by 25 mcg every couple of weeks until symptoms resolve. If your doctor wants you to start with T4-only treatment and you don't get complete resolution of your symptoms, ask to try a T3/T4 combination product.

T3/T4 Combination Products

Some products contain both T3 and T4, in various ratios. Armour Thyroid, the most popular of these products, contains about 80 percent T4 and 20 percent T3, with small amounts of T2 and T1 as well. Other, similar glandular products are also available, such a Naturethroid, Westhroid, and Bio-Throid. There are also synthetic T3/T4 combination products, such as liotrix (Thyrolar).

Dr. Broda Barnes, an early pioneer in thyroid research, treated thousands of people with hypothyroidism in the 1960s and 1970s. He generally used Armour Thyroid and suggested the following guidelines for finding the right dose: Children over six should start at 30 mg, teenagers and adults at 60 mg, and very large adults at 120 mg. He observed that most of his patients noticed a change in their symptoms within the first month or two. If all symptoms didn't resolve after two months, he suggested reevaluating the dose and usually increased doses for teenagers by 30 mg and those for adults by 60 mg. He repeated this increase as necessary until all symptoms were resolved at the lowest possible dose. He said that most of his adult patients required no more than 120 mg, and that only occasionally did people require doses as high as 240 mg (Barnes and Galton 1976). This information is interesting as anecdotal data, but you will obviously need to work with your doctor to assess your individual requirements and optimal dosage level.

T3-Only Products

Some doctors are more comfortable adding a synthetic T3-only drug to their patient's T4 therapy if the person doesn't get complete relief on T4 alone, rather than using a glandular product. This can be a good solution for some people, but it's important to get the right dose of T3, as it acts much more quickly and also breaks down more quickly, having a half-life of about seven hours (as opposed to the seven-day half-life of T4). Because it acts so quickly, it has a pronounced stimulatory effect. Taking too much can trigger symptoms of hyperthyroidism, such as a rapid pulse, an overly strong heartbeat, heart palpitations, nervousness, tremors, feeling too hot or clammy, night sweats, and insomnia (for a more comprehensive list, see the text box later in this chapter).

New research suggests that diseases such as fibromyalgia and chronic fatigue syndrome may respond well to higher-dose T3 therapy alone. It's thought that these diseases may be caused by peripheral thyroid resistance, a condition in which your body becomes less responsive to thyroid hormone action. This condition has been shown to respond well to slowly increasing doses of T3 (Lowe 2000). Another condition that appears to respond well to T3-only therapy is extremely elevated levels of reverse T3. In this situation, adding more T4 could result in additional conversion to more reverse T3, further blocking the body's ability to use whatever T3 is present. Because of T3's short half-life and stimulatory effects, most doctors who use this therapy prescribe multiple smaller doses throughout the day, instead of just one daily dose. The most common T3 drug is liothyronine (Cytomel).

THE INS AND OUTS OF THYROID HORMONE THERAPY

Thyroid hormone therapy is a completely individual process. There is no way to know what the right dose is for any given person without a process of trial and error. In truth, tests results offer only minimal help in establishing your proper dose and managing your ongoing therapy. And all too often, people gradually increase to an optimal dose that resolves all their symptoms only to have their doctor reduce the dose if subsequent blood tests show a "low" TSH level. As you might guess, this lowered dose generally results in a return of symptoms. If this happens, you may need to be assertive with your doctor about maintaining the optimal dose that succeeded in resolving all your symptoms. A lower dose would be appropriate, however, if you begin to experience any symptoms of hyperthyroidism, such as those listed in the text box (as long as they aren't caused by an underlying adrenal deficiency).

If you start taking thyroid hormones or increase your dose, you should keep the following symptoms of excess thyroid activity in mind. If you develop any of these symptoms after starting thyroid hormone therapy, it's important to notify your doctor right away and then work with him or her to adjust your dosage:

- Breathlessness

- Fatigue

- Heart palpitations and/or fast heart rate

- Heat intolerance

- Increased bowel movements

- Insomnia

- Irritability

- Muscle weakness

- Nervousness

- Overly warm, moist skin

- Trembling hands

To ensure that the information from lab tests is as relevant and helpful as possible, never take your thyroid medication before your blood test on the day the blood is drawn, as this will result in inaccurate readings. It's best to take your last dose twenty-four hours prior to your test.

Most doctors are leery about high thyroid hormone doses (particularly when using T3 as well as T4) due to concerns about osteoporosis and heart disease. Osteoporosis appears to be a fairly nonexistent risk unless the dosage is actually causing hyperthyroidism. To prevent your doctor from feeling he or she is shouldering any unnecessary liability in this regard, you can offer to take a simple N-telopeptide (NTx) urine test. This test determines whether you're losing bone faster than you're rebuilding it due to elevated metabolism.

The only heart-related concern with thyroid hormone therapy is in the case of a significantly damaged or weakened heart. If you have any history of heart disease or heart attack, you should work with your doctor to thoroughly evaluate your heart function before starting thyroid hormone therapy. On the other hand, clinical studies have shown that low T3 levels are a "strong predictor of death in cardiac patients and might be directly implicated in the poor prognosis of cardiac patients" (Iervasi et al. 2003, 708), so thyroid hormone therapy may be very beneficial to most of these people. The best course of action is to be extremely cautious, working with your doctor to start at very low doses, and increasing the dose slowly.

This is actually a good idea for everyone, no matter what thyroid medication you and your doctor decide to use. If your metabolism has been suppressed for some time, it will take a while for your body to adjust to the new, higher demands placed on it by an increased metabolic rate.

TREATING HYPOTHYROIDISM WHEN YOU ALSO HAVE ADRENAL FATIGUE

In light of the close relationship between your thyroid and your adrenals, an issue you need to be aware of is the effect supplemental thyroid hormones have on your adrenal function. Here's how it works: Thyroid hormone supplementation increases your metabolism, making greater demands on systems throughout your body. If you have adrenal fatigue, this will put extra strain on your adrenal glands to increase their production of hormones. If your adrenals are on their last legs, they'll get increasingly exhausted, making you feel worse and worse (more tired, achy, and so on). When this happens, people often assume that thyroid therapy is making them feel worse rather than better, so they stop taking thyroid medication, depriving themselves of the chance to finally feel better and regain their health.

If you start taking thyroid hormones and either get very little benefit or notice symptoms of hyperthyroidism on a very low dose, it's likely that your problem is insufficient adrenal function. (Chapter 9 discusses this in detail.) If this happens, make sure you work with your doctor to evaluate whether low adrenal function is the cause.

Alternately, you may notice that you feel great for a while after starting thyroid medication but then start to feel worse in a month or two as you increase your dose. This is often because your liver, stimulated by your increased metabolic rate, begins to clear stores of cortisol from your body much more quickly than your adrenals can replace it, leading eventually to a shortage of cortisol. It's important to measure your cortisol levels after two to three months of thyroid hormone therapy. It's not uncommon to see levels at 50 percent of what they were when you started, revealing a hidden adrenal deficiency.

What to Expect as You Raise Your Dose

You may feel good as soon as you start thyroid hormone therapy and continue to get more benefit as you increase your dose until you arrive at your optimal dose. However, most of us experience an ebbing and flowing of symptoms as we start taking thyroid hormones. Generally, for people starting thyroid therapy for the first time, doctors begin with 30 mg of Armour Thyroid or 25 to 50 mcg of levothyroxine (Synthroid). Because these initial doses are so low, you may not notice a difference until you begin to increase your dose.

If you do have increased feelings of well-being and some resolution of your symptoms but this fades after just a couple of days or a week, don't panic. This just means that your dose is too low, and now that your body has adjusted its metabolism up a notch, it wants even more thyroid hormones. Your doctor will generally continue to raise your dose in 15 to 30 mg increments for Armour Thyroid and 25 mcg increments for Synthroid. Working closely with your doctor during this process is very important in resolving your symptoms as quickly and painlessly as possible—and in making sure you don't end up with hyperthyroidism. Dosage levels that are too high can set back the process a bit, as you will then need to lower your dose until the overstimulation subsides, adding another trial-and-error phase to the process of determining your optimum dose. It's much better to just go slowly and steadily so you don't suddenly place excessive demands on your body and its depressed metabolism.

A note of caution: If your blood tests weren't obviously indicative of hypothyroidism and your doctor is giving you a trial course of hormone therapy to see if thyroid dysfunction could be causing your symptoms, be very vigilant about assessing whether you actually feel worse after starting thyroid hormone therapy. If the tips in the troubleshooting section at the end of this chapter don't resolve any symptoms that have gotten worse, such as hair loss or increased fatigue, you can assume that thyroid therapy isn't the right solution for your situation. And if you don't have hypothyroidism, you should *never* use supplemental thyroid hormones for weight loss. If thyroid dysfunction isn't the root cause of your weight problem, supplementation will result in side effects such as heart palpitations and nervousness, but not weight loss.

Dosing Tips

Studies have shown that the key to successful thyroid therapy is to take your medication consistently. In other words, you should take it around the same time and in the same way each day (for example, without food, chewed or swallowed, and so on). Changing these variables may result in inconsistent results.

Most people report good results when they take their thyroid medication first thing in the morning, at least half an hour before they eat anything. A recent small study found that taking T4-only medication at bedtime resulted in higher free T4 levels and lower TSH levels than when the same dose was taken in the morning (Bolk et al. 2007). This may indicate that the medication was better absorbed when taken in the evening. More evidence is needed to confirm these findings, but it may be worth considering if you take your thyroid medication in the morning and aren't experiencing complete resolution of your symptoms.

However, be aware that these findings may not apply to a T3/T4 combination therapy or T3-only therapy. In fact, taking T3 in the evening may not be a good idea, as it has a more stimulating effect and could interfere with sleep. Some doctors recommend that people take T3 thyroid medications in more than one daily dose.

Switching from One Type of Product to Another

If you've tried a T4-only product and it hasn't resolved all of your symptoms, you may be interested in switching to Armour Thyroid or another T3/T4 combination product. This could be very helpful, but you need to work closely with your doctor when changing medications. If you go this route, there are several things to keep in mind.

First, let's look at the math involved in determining an equivalent dose of Armour Thyroid. A dose of 60 mg, or 1 grain, contains 9 mcg of T3 and 38 mcg of T4. To make the conversion between a T4 drug and a combination drug, doctors take into consideration that T3 is approximately four times as potent as T4. Therefore, the 9 mcg of T3 is multiplied by 4 and added to the 38 mcg of T4: 9 mcg x 4 = 36 + 38 = 74 mcg of T4. However, this is just an approximation. The actual effect will differ from woman to woman, which is one reason you'll need to work closely with your doctor during the process of switching from one type of product to another. Your doctor can help assess your symptoms and whether you're improving, and might also want to order follow-up lab tests for more data on how you're responding.

Another consideration with making the switch is that T3 works much more rapidly than T4, so you need to make sure the new medication doesn't become too stimulating. As mentioned, many doctors recommend taking smaller doses throughout the day to help with this problem. Also, T3 is generally better absorbed than T4, as the absorption of T4 is more affected by things like how much you've eaten, your age, and your ability to absorb substances, which can be impacted by gut health and other issues.

Protect Your Thyroid Medication

Thyroid hormones are delicate and subject to degradation. To maintain fairly constant levels in your body and not yo-yo up and down, you should keep a couple of safeguards in mind. First, try to make sure that the product you buy hasn't been subjected to extreme variations in temperature and moisture on the pharmacy shelf. Armour Thyroid is generally shipped to pharmacies in thousand-pill containers. This container is then opened periodically to dispense prescriptions. Depending on the weather, the conditions in the pharmacy, and so on, the thyroid drug can lose potency.

Another consideration is shelf life; the longer the container sits on the shelf and the older the medication is, the less potent it's likely to be. Of course, you usually won't know how long the container has been on the shelf or what the conditions in the pharmacy have been. The easiest way to ensure high quality is to request that the pharmacist get you an unopened hundred-pill container of Armour Thyroid from Forest Labs, the manufacturer of Armour Thyroid. If your pharmacist can't do this, make sure you ask what the date is on their container, as small pharmacies may have the thousand-pill containers on their shelves for a long period of time. Forest Labs has recently come out with individual blister packaging for Armour Thyroid, which may ensure quality, but this has not yet been confirmed by independent testing.

How you store your medication is also important. Store it at room temperature in a place where the temperature is fairly constant. Keep the top tightly closed to seal out moisture. When you fly, you shouldn't put your thyroid medicine in your checked luggage, as it would be subjected to huge temperature variations in the baggage compartment of the airplane.

Interactions with Other Substances

Many drugs, and some vitamins and minerals, can interact with thyroid medication. They often interfere with absorption and can be the cause for less than satisfactory results.

MINERAL SUPPLEMENTS

Iron and calcium can interfere with absorption and utilization of supplemental thyroid hormones. These minerals should be taken two to three hours away from your thyroid medication. Don't overlook less obvious supplemental sources, such as multivitamins, orange juice, and other foods that may be fortified with iron or calcium.

DRUGS

Certain drugs have been proven to impair the effectiveness of thyroid hormone therapy. Because new drugs come on the market so often, and because ongoing research will reveal more about drugs and their interactions, it's important to view this list as a starting point. If you're taking other medications in addition to thyroid hormones, be sure to ask your doctor or pharmacist about any possible interactions:

- Fluoroquinolone antibiotics such as ciprofloxacin (Cipro, Ciproxin and Ciprobay) are known to interfere with thyroid therapy (Cooper et al. 2005), perhaps by decreasing absorption of thyroid drugs. Ciprofloxacin is primarily used to treat pneumonia, urinary tract infections, and sexually transmitted diseases. It seems that it doesn't have this effect when taken at least six hours apart from thyroid medication, so take it as far apart from your thyroid therapy as possible.

- Estrogen-only hormone replacement therapy or the use of birth control pills may require an increased dose of thyroid hormones (Arafah 2001).

- The antidepressant medications sertraline (Zoloft), paroxetine (Paxil), and fluoxetine (Prozac) can make thyroid medication either more or less effective, depending on the individual. Especially close monitoring is needed when starting or stopping one of these drugs while on thyroid medication.

- Sucralfate (Carafate), an ulcer medication, can interfere with the absorption of thyroid hormones.

- The cholesterol-lowering drugs cholestyramine (Questran) and colestipol (Cholestid) can also affect absorption of your thyroid medication.

In addition, any drug that affects your thyroid may impair the effectiveness of thyroid therapy. For example, sulfa and antihistamine drugs inhibit the thyroid's uptake of iodine. For more details, see "Medications," in chapter 5.

TROUBLESHOOTING

Ideally, when you start on thyroid hormone therapy you'd experience a rapid resolution of symptoms and few or no problems. But as we know, the real world doesn't always work that way. If you have difficulties at first, don't get discouraged. The troubleshooting tips below will help you identify and solve some of the most common problems.

Because thyroid hormone overdose and cortisol deficiency are possible causes of many of the problems discussed below, here are some pointers on these two concerns. To determine whether excessive amounts of supplemental thyroid hormones are causing the problem, look for other signs of an excessive stimulation, including overheating, nervousness, and insomnia listed on page 84.

Cortisol deficiency, or adrenal fatigue, can make you intolerant of thyroid hormone therapy to the extent that you may develop symptoms of hyperthyroidism very quickly. If this is the case, you must address adrenal deficiencies in order to be successful with your thyroid therapy. To determine if cortisol deficiency is a problem, look for other signs of low cortisol levels, such as fatigue, low blood pressure, allergies, and irritability. (See chapter 9 for a detailed discussion of adrenal function, along with a symptoms evaluation, some simple tests you can do at home, and details on lab tests and treatment of cortisol deficiency.)

The following troubleshooting suggestions are made by Dr. Thierry Hertoghe in *The Hormone Handbook* (2006), his hormone therapy guide for doctors. For each problem, potential causes are listed from most to least common.

Problem: Signs of cardiac stimulation, such as heart palpitations even at low doses	
Possible Causes	**Solutions**
Cortisol deficiency	Correct a cortisol deficiency with adrenal support.
Thyroid hormone overdose	Work with your doctor to lower your dose of thyroid hormones.

Problem: Headaches	
Possible Causes	**Solutions**
Thyroid hormone overdose	Work with your doctor to lower your dose of thyroid hormones.
Cortisol deficiency	Correct a cortisol deficiency with adrenal support.
Exposure to toxic chemicals	Consider blood tests to determine whether you have excessive levels of chemical pollutants such as mercury, cadmium, and other heavy metals.
Low estrogen	Measure levels of estrogen to detect any deficiency and work with your doctor to correct it with supplemental bioidentical estrogen.

Problem: Diarrhea	
Possible Causes	**Solutions**
Thyroid hormone overdose	Work with your doctor to lower your dose of thyroid hormones.
Cortisol deficiency	Correct a cortisol deficiency with adrenal support.
Excessive magnesium or iron supplementation	Stop taking magnesium or iron supplements, or lower your dosage.
Food intolerance or allergy	Avoid foods that are problematic for you, and consider testing to determine whether other foods may be causing inflammation or allergic reaction.
Yeast or bacterial infections	Treat any intestinal yeast overgrowth or bacterial infections.

Problem: Symptoms of low estrogen levels, such as hot flashes, loss of breast tissue, a pale face, headaches, absent or very light periods, and shortened menstrual cycles lasting less than twenty-one days	
Possible Causes	**Solutions**
Thyroid hormones accelerated metabolism of estrogen, clearing it from your body quickly and causing a shortage.	Take supplemental estrogen and progesterone. If this doesn't correct the problem, try a lower dose of thyroid hormones.

Problem: Failure to lose excess weight while dieting	
Possible Causes	**Solutions**
Both low-calorie and high-protein/low-carb diets slow conversion of T4 to T3, so you may not have enough T3 to increase your metabolism and help you lose weight.	Increase your thyroid dose by 15 to 30 percent after a week of this type of diet if you have limited results. Another alternative is to use a T3/T4 combination drug not a T4-only drug.

WHAT'S NEXT?

Finding the optimal form and dose of thyroid hormones may involve trying several different products, dosages, and schedules for taking the medication. The process can take several months—yet another reason why it's so important to find a doctor you're comfortable with. You need to find a doctor who will not only guide you through the medical aspects, but also encourage and support you through this sometimes frustrating process. Invest the time up front to interview different doctors until you find the right partner. It will pay off in huge returns by helping you resolve your symptoms as quickly as possible.

An effective treatment program can go a long way toward resolving your symptoms. However, underlying lifestyle factors such as poor diet or lack of exercise may have contributed to the problem, and can perpetuate it as well. In the next chapter, we'll take a look at ways you can support your thyroid function—and your overall health.

KEY POINTS

🖐 Figuring out optimal doses of thyroid hormones should be an individualized process. There is no way to know what the right dose is for any given person without a process of trial and error while keeping a careful eye on symptoms. Test results offer little help in finding your ideal dose or managing your ongoing therapy.

🖐 Thyroid hormone products include T4-only drugs such as levothyroxine (Synthroid); T3-only drugs such as liothyronine (Cytomel), which can be used alone or with a T4 drug; and T3/T4 combination products in both synthetic forms and in the form of glandular extracts, notably Armour Thyroid.

🖐 Picking the right thyroid medication for your individual needs is critical to successful thyroid hormone therapy. T4 alone may not resolve your symptoms if you're unable to convert T4 to T3 because of stress, diet, or illness, or because of excessive production of reverse T3. The deciding factor in whether to use a T4-only product or a T3/T4 combination drug should be your level of free T3 or your response to T4-only therapy.

🖐 Many drugs can interact with thyroid medication and be the cause of less than satisfactory results from thyroid therapy.

CHAPTER 8

Other Ways to Support
Your Thyroid Function

It's critical to support your thyroid and overall endocrine health by eating a good diet, making wise lifestyle choices, and avoiding exposure to toxic chemicals. Years of low thyroid function (and possibly other hormone deficiencies as well), a poor diet, drinking too much alcohol, lack of exercise, exposure to toxins, or too much stress can take a toll on your metabolism. Depending on the nature of the insult, the damage can take years to develop, or it may occur in just a few months.

Not surprisingly, the symptoms of metabolic damage are much the same as symptoms of low thyroid function, as both indicate that your metabolic rate is inadequate for your body's needs. And likewise, both your thyroid function and your metabolism will benefit from some basic changes in your lifestyle and diet. It's easier than you think—and an important first step in ensuring a future free from many of the diseases and conditions we generally associate with aging. There's no need for us to assume we'll inevitably end up with dementia, obesity, chronic pain, heart disease, neurological disorders, cancer, or brittle, broken bones.

This chapter will take a close look at lifestyle choices that can help you rebuild your metabolic function, but all of this information can be distilled into a few commonsense pointers:

- Reduce or manage stress.

- Improve your diet and nutrition.

- Get enough rest and sleep.

   🌿   Stay active.

   🌿   Avoid exposure to toxic chemicals.

DIET AND NUTRITION

The right kind of diet is extremely important if you have low thyroid function—or even if you're simply trying to optimize your thyroid health. Because hypothyroidism prevents you from absorbing nutrients well, what you eat is especially critical when you have this condition. Eating a balanced diet and taking supplements as needed, will go a long way toward helping rebuild your damaged metabolism.

The Best Balance

As is true in so many other areas of life, balance is the key to choosing foods that support your thyroid, as well as the rest of your endocrine system. You need the right balance of protein, fats, and complex carbohydrates. Many nutritionists believe the optimum breakdown is about 26 percent fats, 37 percent complex carbohydrates (primarily in the form of vegetables and whole grains), and 37 percent protein in terms of calories consumed daily. It's a good idea to try to eat all three—fats, complex carbohydrates and protein—at every meal, as this will keep your blood sugar levels fairly even. Too many carbohydrates and too few fats cause swings in blood sugar levels. But again, balance is the key: Since your brain uses only carbohydrates for fuel, not protein or fats, consuming enough complex carbohydrates is also critical.

Fat has been demonized for the last twenty years, in part due to its high calorie content. When calorie counting came into fashion, it was thought that fat would cause more weight gain than protein or carbohydrates (since each gram of fat has 9 calories, as opposed to 4 calories for each gram of protein or carbohydrate). Further, it was believed that saturated fats, which are high in cholesterol, would somehow stick to the blood vessels and cause heart disease. This belief led many of us to avoid saturated fats and switch to smaller amounts of unsaturated fats; for example, substituting margarine for butter. At the same time, we embraced carbohydrates with a vengeance and ate lots of pasta, potatoes, rice, and bread. Subsequently, research has proven that excess refined carbohydrates, such as sugar and white flour, are also culprits in elevated cholesterol levels and heart disease (Liu et al. 2000). In addition, adequate amounts of good-quality fats are critical for good thyroid function.

"Good-quality" is an important qualifier. You should avoid trans fats and hydrogenated oils at all costs, because of their toxic effects on health. Saturated fats, such as butter and coconut oil, are fine in moderation. And because they're more stable at high heat, they're good choices for cooking with, as are monounsaturated fats, such as olive oil. And of course omega-3 fatty acids, so abundant in flaxseed oil and coldwater fish, are now widely acclaimed for their health benefits. Most of us could probably use more of these healthy fats in our diet. But steer clear of heating flaxseed oil (and other oils high in polyunsaturated fats), as they're easily damaged.

More recently, carbohydrates, too, have been vilified. However, the situation isn't so simple. As with fats, quality is critical, and it's especially important to distinguish between two different types of carbohydrates—simple and complex—and between whole foods and refined, processed foods.

Simple carbohydrates are made up of single sugar molecules or two sugar molecules joined together. They're found in many foods, from fruits to milk, and, of course, refined sugar, and are rapidly absorbed into the bloodstream. Complex carbohydrates are also made up of sugars, but the sugar molecules are strung together to form longer, more complex chains, so they're absorbed into the bloodstream more slowly. Plus, many foods high in complex carbohydrates, such as whole grains, beans, vegetables, and peas, contain a good amount of fiber, which adds bulk that causes them to be converted into blood sugar even more slowly. This keeps blood sugar levels steadier and therefore results in reduced, slower insulin release.

However, many of these benefits are lost when foods are refined and processed, as in white rice, white flour, sugar, and so on. Processing strips them of their fiber-rich outer covering and, in the case of grains, the nutrient-rich germ. It also causes them to convert to blood sugar, or glucose, much more quickly. These foods are very damaging to your body, as many of their valuable vitamins and minerals have been removed, along with the enzymes necessary for digestion. This forces your body to rob itself of these substances in order to process refined carbohydrates, so they have a net negative effect on the body, rather than a positive one.

Beware of Fad Diets

Fad diets are a fact of life in our increasingly overweight modern society: the high-protein/low-carb diet, the low-protein/high-carb diet, the low-fat diet, the starvation diet, and endless variations on these themes. Millions of Americans can testify to the fact that these diets don't work in the long run, though they often believe it's an issue of willpower. In truth, this problem has more to do with our biochemistry, as many of these diets compromise thyroid function.

One of the biggest problems with all of these diets that have been so popular in recent years is the lack of balance they involve. Eating a greater proportion of any one type of food, whether it's fat, carbs, or protein, will deprive you of necessary amounts of one or more of the others, and all are required for your thyroid to function well.

As previously discussed, simple calorie restriction is problematic, as well. The depressing biological reality we encounter all too quickly is that when we cut our food intake too radically, the body thinks it's in a famine situation and produces a lot more reverse T3 to slow metabolism. This allows us to survive until food becomes plentiful again, but it doesn't result in weight loss. It simply results in various symptoms of hypothyroidism, like hair loss and feeling cold and tired.

Another problem is that the muscle cells can store only so much of the excessive amounts of glucose released when you eat refined carbohydrates. Once they get full, your body has to release more insulin to try to manage the remaining glucose. This causes your blood sugar level to drop suddenly, so you end up craving caffeine, sugar, and simple carbs, which just perpetuates the cycle and puts you on the road to type 2 diabetes. If you're eating lots of refined carbohydrates and experiencing cravings you can't seem to control, you should seriously consider trying to cut them out entirely for a period of time to normalize your blood sugar and insulin levels. You'll find it gets easier every day, and eventually the cravings should stop.

A Few Other Guidelines

One simple rule to follow is to eat foods as close to their natural state as possible. In terms of carbohydrates, this means choosing whole grains and whole-grain products rather than refined carbohydrates. It's also best to choose organic foods whenever possible; this will help you avoid all of those endocrine-disrupting chemicals that non-organic produce is treated with.

There are a few foods that people with hypothyroidism should avoid, since they contain goitrogens, naturally occurring substances that suppress thyroid function, such as vegetables like cabbage, kale, rutabaga, turnips, and soybeans. You can find exhaustive lists of these foods online, but the truth is, balance is once again the key. These foods are generally very good for you, so if you eat them in moderation, you should be fine. Another problem with soybeans, however, is that they can interfere with intestinal absorption of iodine, which will also impair thyroid function. In the 1950s, babies who were given soymilk because they were allergic to cow's milk developed iodine deficiency. The problem was resolved by adding iodine to soymilk baby formulas.

Timing of meals is also important. If possible, you should eat smaller, more frequent meals rather than three big meals a day. This will help keep your blood sugar even and allow your metabolism to plug along at a steady pace. Plus, blood sugar swings can contribute to fatigue and brain fog, symptoms you'd probably rather avoid.

The Bottom Line

All of the ever-changing nutritional info out there can be confusing, and even once you understand the basics outlined above, you may wonder what an optimum diet really is. Here are some basic dietary recommendations you should try to follow whenever possible:

- Restrict your consumption of refined carbohydrates and sugar. Eat complex (whole-grain) carbohydrates instead. This is important for both overall health and weight loss.

- Eat lots of fruits and vegetables and other high-fiber foods to keep your intestines clean and encourage the growth of friendly bacteria in your digestive tract.

- Eat moderate servings (roughly the size of your palm) of lean protein, from both animal and plant sources. Fish and poultry are the leanest animal proteins. Nuts and beans are good plant sources of protein.

- Choose healthy sources of fat such as nuts, nut butters, avocados, olive oil, and other vegetable oils (including in salad dressings). Make sure to include plenty of oils high in omega-3s and to stay away from all trans fats.

- Limit your consumption of processed food products and fast food. These are often loaded with sugar and chemicals.

- Limit your consumption of soft drinks, as they can leach magnesium and calcium from your bones. (And never drink diet soft drinks because of added chemicals!)

- Drink plenty of chlorine- and fluoride-free water; eight glasses a day is the recommended minimum.

- Try and eat organic foods whenever possible to reduce your exposure to chemicals that can affect your thyroid and other endocrine glands.

Vitamin and Mineral Supplements

Even with a healthy whole foods diet with lots of organic foods, you may be deficient in certain nutrients. A good preventative measure is to take a good multivitamin and mineral supplement. Talk to the expert at your local vitamin shop or natural food store for recommendations.

The Importance of Iodine

The main metabolic function of iodine is to enable the thyroid to synthesize, store, and secrete thyroid hormones. About 75 percent of the iodine you consume goes to your thyroid gland, with the rest going to the gut, breasts, stomach, bones, connective tissues, extracellular fluids, and nasal secretions.

In the United States, iodine is added to most table salt to ensure we get enough of this important mineral in our diet. The amount of iodine currently recommended is 150 mcg, which you can get from just over 1/2 teaspoon of iodized salt. Pregnant and breastfeeding women require more: 157 mcg daily and 200 mcg daily, respectively. Fruits and vegetables grown in coastal regions with iodine-rich soil are also good sources of iodine, as are seafood and seaweeds, such as kelp.

If you have hypothyroidism, it's important to get enough iodine in your diet, but be cautious with iodine supplements. Excess iodine intake can actually reduce thyroid activity in people who have compromised thyroid function, particularly those with Hashimoto's thyroiditis. Watch for signs of hypothyroidism if you do supplement it, and be aware that it can further damage your thyroid gland.

OTHER CRITICAL SUPPLEMENTS FOR THYROID SUPPORT

To make and utilize thyroid hormones, you also need adequate levels of the following nutrients:

- Calcium
- Chromium
- Coenzyme Q10
- Copper
- Folic acid
- Iron
- Magnesium
- Manganese
- Omega-3 fatty acids
- Selenium
- Tyrosine
- Vitamin A
- Vitamin B (including B_1, B_2, B_3, B_5, B_6, and B_{12})
- Vitamin C
- Vitamin E
- Zinc

LIFESTYLE CONSIDERATIONS

There are some basic, commonsense things you can incorporate into your lifestyle to support your thyroid function—and your entire endocrine system. Let's take a look at some of the important ones.

Get enough rest and sleep. Try to get seven and a half to eight and a half hours of sleep each night. The bare minimum for most women is somewhere around five hours, but many of us suffer if we sleep less than eight.

Stay active. It may seem counterintuitive, but physical activity can actually increase your energy level. Plus, it's one of the best ways to reduce stress and can even normalize adrenal function, lowering cortisol levels if they're too high or raising them if they're too low. If you don't currently have an exercise routine, the best way to come up with one that you'll stick to is to find something you enjoy doing that fits your schedule and lifestyle. Something as simple as a daily walk can be incredibly beneficial, not just for your thyroid function, but also to help stave off depression, heart disease, diabetes, and many other chronic diseases.

Reduce stress. Take a close look at what's causing stress in your life and consider whether you can make any changes so that you experience less of it. And because we can't realistically avoid all stress, take the time to learn stress management skills so you can handle it in a more healthy way. A key strategy is to participate in activities that reduce your stress level. This is different for every woman. Whether it's going out to lunch with friends, meditating, praying, or simply watching soap operas with your feet up, make sure you take time out of your undoubtedly busy schedule to enjoy stress-relieving activities regularly. If time is a big factor for you, keep in mind that exercise is a highly effective way to reduce your stress level. By making time for physical activity, you'll be killing two birds with one stone—something all of us multitaskers should appreciate.

Avoid alcohol, stimulants, and other harmful substances. In your quest for optimal thyroid and hormonal health, there are some obvious substances to avoid. The first and most obvious is alcohol. Because it's fermented, it can lead to yeast overgrowth. It also can damage the thyroid gland directly when consumed in excess. It's also important to avoid caffeine and other stimulants, which raise your level of adrenaline and cause it to remain in your body for longer periods. This will deplete your body of important biochemicals and damage your metabolism even further.

TRY TO AVOID HEAVY METALS AND HARMFUL CHEMICALS

Avoiding all toxic chemicals is obviously important, but this is often easier said than done. These days we are surrounded by harmful substances, including heavy metals and other toxic industrial pollutants, chemicals in everything from household cleansers to fabrics to body care items, and even seemingly benign food additives.

Heavy Metals

Exposure to heavy metals causes a complex cascade of effects in our bodies, including activating the immune system. This can lead to problems with hypothalamus, pituitary, thyroid, and adrenal functions. The metals that most commonly cause immune reactivity are nickel, mercury, chromium, cobalt, and palladium.

The U.S. Centers for Disease Control ranks toxic metals as the number one environmental health threat to children, with mercury, lead, arsenic, and cadmium all ranked in the top eight most toxic; chromium is also high on the list (Agency for Toxic Substances and Disease Registry 1999). These toxic metals can cause fatigue, pain, sleep disturbances, severe psychological symptoms such as depression, and gastrointestinal and neurological problems.

It's been well-known for years that mercury disrupts the endocrine system and can result in severe damage to both this system and the nervous system. Studies have shown that mercury causes hypothyroidism, autoimmune thyroiditis, and damage to thyroid RNA, and also impairs conversion of T4 to T3 (Sterzl et al. 2006). It blocks thyroid hormone production by interfering with iodine utilization and prevents normal action of thyroid hormones. This results in inadequate thyroid stimulation even though your thyroid hormone levels may appear to be normal. Mercury also blocks your body's ability to effectively use vitamins B_6 and B_{12}, calcium, magnesium, and zinc, which are all important to thyroid function.

Mercury rapidly crosses the blood-brain barrier and is stored first in the hypothalamus, pituitary, and occipital lobe (responsible for visual processing). It damages these areas, as well as the blood-brain barrier itself, enabling other toxic metals and substances to penetrate the brain. It's also stored in, and damages, the thyroid. The hormones most often affected by mercury are thyroid hormones, insulin, estrogen, testosterone, and adrenaline. Major sources of mercury exposure are mercury amalgam dental fillings and thimerosal, a mercury-based preservative found in vaccinations and other medicines.

Lead can also be toxic to your thyroid gland and in clinical studies has been shown to raise TSH levels and lower T3 (Singh et al. 2000). Lead has widely known adverse effects on the nervous system. It can also damage the endocrine system and may seriously affect reproductive function, as well as organs and tissues.

We're exposed to cadmium, an industrial pollutant, from a wide variety of sources. It's found in auto exhaust, industrial waste, cigarette smoke, sewage sludge, batteries, and fertilizers. Both drinking water and food crops may also be contaminated with cadmium. High levels of cadmium can cause not only thyroid abnormalities but also kidney and liver damage and anemia.

If you have symptoms of hypothyroidism, it's important to ask your doctor to measure your levels of toxic metals, as they can damage your thyroid gland, your entire endocrine system, and your nervous system. The best way to do this is with something known as a urine challenge test. For this test, you take a pill containing a substance that has an affinity for binding to heavy metals. This causes them to be excreted in your urine, where their levels can be measured. If they're elevated, you should work with your doctor to reduce levels of toxic heavy metals in your body.

Harmful Chemicals

Toxic chemicals and pollutants enter our bodies all the time, and we continually eliminate them naturally through the kidneys and colon. But many toxins are able to imitate our natural biochemicals (including hormones) and get into our cell walls. The toxins that mimic our hormones fit into hormone receptor sites on cell surfaces and hamper the body's ability to eliminate them. This also blocks hormones from binding with those sites and performing their normal functions and leads to cell and tissue damage.

Iodine falls into the class of elements known as halogens, which also includes fluorine, chlorine, and bromine (and the obscure astatine). Because these elements share certain characteristics, they react similarly. As a result, fluorine, chlorine, and bromine can bind with iodine receptors in the thyroid gland, which results in decreased production of thyroid hormones. Unfortunately, we're awash in a sea of halogens and compounds that contain them: fluorine in tap water and toothpastes (in the form of fluoride); chlorine in tap water, sanitizers, cleansers, and plastics; and bromine in some bread products, brominated vegetable oil (an emulsifier added to certain soft drinks), hot tub cleansers, plastics, personal care products, certain medications, fabric dyes, and fire retardants. Fluorine, chlorine, and bromine have also been implicated in other thyroid diseases, not just hypothyroidism. This includes autoimmune diseases and even thyroid cancer (Malenchenko, Demidchik, and Tadeush 1984). In adequate amounts, iodine will push out excessive fluorine, chlorine, and bromine from your body, making it an excellent natural detoxifier.

Food additives are an often-overlooked cause of toxic chemical exposure. Your thyroid is continually being assaulted by chemicals and hydrogenated oils (trans fats). The process of hydrogenation alters the chemical makeup of fats to give them an extended shelf life. However, this alteration also causes them to disrupt the normal functioning of cells and blocks our utilization of fatty acids, which are critical in thyroid function. Trans fats have been implicated in various other health problems, too, especially heart disease. Fortunately, regulatory agencies and food manufacturers are starting to take notice, so the use of trans fats is beginning to decrease. Some states are getting serious about it. New York has led the way as the first state to ban their use in all restaurants. In the meanwhile, read labels carefully and be aware that these damaging fats are often used in bakery products and fast-food restaurants, where they're used for deep-frying.

REPAIRING METABOLIC DAMAGE

Long-term hypothyroidism, poor diet or lifestyle choices, exposure to toxic chemicals, or a combination of these factors can result in compromised metabolic and immune function. This damage is often manifested in conditions such as allergies, digestion problems, and candida overgrowth. Thyroid hormone therapy will help restore immune function and prevent further damage, but it's important to detect and treat these conditions concurrently, as they can affect your ability to completely resolve your symptoms even with thyroid therapy.

Food Allergies

Some of the most common food allergies we start to see increasing after age thirty are to gluten or wheat, eggs, dairy, shellfish, peanuts, tree nuts, soy, or foods in the nightshade family, such as tomatoes and peppers. Food allergies can cause a variety of symptoms, such as stomach problems, headaches, sinus congestion, fatigue, and even depression. They can also undermine your immune system.

If you suspect you may have food allergies, you should work with your doctor to test them to be sure. Alternatively, you can try cutting out the foods most likely to cause allergies or any foods that seem to cause negative symptoms when you eat them. This trial and error method is simply to stop eating a certain food for seven to ten days—one food group at a time. If you feel better after this period of time, it indicates that you may be allergic to these foods. After you get them out of your system, you should feel much better and see your overall health improve.

Digestion Problems

Indigestion and bowel problems (including irritable bowel syndrome) can be caused by the inability to digest food properly. Inflammation in the GI tract due to deficiencies or imbalances of vitamins, minerals, and hormones often results in decreased production of stomach acid and digestive enzymes. This impairs the body's ability to derive needed nutrients from food, perpetuating the cycle. Using supplemental digestive enzymes and betaine hydrochloride (essentially, stomach acid) will help to increase digestion.

However, treating just the symptoms in this way should only be a stopgap measure. You need to figure out the root cause of your digestion problems, which may be causing damage to your bowel lining. Possibilities include antibiotic use, toxins, poor diet, parasites, and infection. These can all cause your gut wall to become more permeable to undigested food, toxins, microbes, or waste products (Martin 1995). Using probiotics will help balance your intestinal flora and heal your intestinal lining, which can result in better digestive function and absorption of nutrients. Low thyroid or adrenal function, or other endocrine disorders, can be at the root of all of these problems, so you must also test for and treat these deficiencies in order to get lasting results.

Candida or Yeast Overgrowth

Candida albicans is a fungus that belongs to the yeast family. As mentioned in chapter 5, you can have it in various parts of your body, including your digestive tract. The amount of yeast in your intestinal tract is controlled by benign microbes. If these microbes are destroyed, generally by antibiotic use, candida growth can get out of control and release toxins, damaging your central nervous system and your immune system. Some of the conditions that have been linked to an overgrowth of candida include confusion, hyperactivity, aggression, short attention span, lethargy, irritability, headaches, constipation, bloating, gas pains, stomachaches, fatigue, and depression. Candida overgrowth can also damage your thyroid.

Mitochondrial Repair

Mitochondria, the energy generators in our cells, can be damaged due to a variety of causes, a primary one being long-term hypothyroidism. It's important to support your body in resuscitating your mitochondria in conjunction with thyroid hormone therapy. Several supplements may be helpful, including acetyl-L-carnitine, carnosine, taurine, R-lipoic acid, and N-acetylcysteine.

Easy Candida Test

Here's a simple test to see if you may have an overgrowth of candida: When
up in the morning, before brushing your teeth or eating, generate some saliva and then
enough into a clear glass of water to cover the surface. Observe the water periodically for up
to ten minutes for the following signs:

> *k* Strings coming down from your saliva (like jellyfish tentacles)

> *k* The water becoming cloudy

> *k* The saliva sinking to the bottom of the glass

Healthy saliva will simply float on top of the water, so if you have any of these signs,
you may have candida overgrowth. If testing or symptoms show candida overgrowth, you
should eliminate all sugar and refined carbohydrates from your diet, as well as anything
containing yeast, such as bread. This will starve the candida. Work with your doctor to find
the best treatment to resolve it, which may involve using one of the prescription antifungal
drugs such as fluconazole (Diflucan) or nystatin (Nystan), or over-the-counter caprylic acid.
You should also always test your adrenal function if you find you have candida overgrowth,
as low adrenal function is often one of the causes.

WHAT'S NEXT?

Supplemental thyroid hormones, a good diet, and a healthy lifestyle can go a long way to resolving
your symptoms of hypothyroidism. However, as mentioned several times, compromised adrenal
function can impair your thyroid health and even prevent you from fully responding to thyroid
hormones (both supplemental and your body's own supply). For treatment of hypothyroidism to
be effective, adrenal problems must be assessed and treated at the same time. The next chapter
provides a full discussion of this important topic, along with a symptom evaluation to help you
determine whether adrenal complications are an issue for you.

KEY POINTS

🐾 Rebuilding your metabolic function is a priority if you have low thyroid function. Key strategies include improving your diet and nutrition, getting enough rest and sleep, staying active, reducing or managing stress, and avoiding toxic substances.

🐾 You need the right balance of high-quality protein, fats, and complex carbohydrates to best support your thyroid function and overall health. A good target goal is 26 percent fats, 37 percent complex carbohydrates (primarily vegetables and whole grains), and 37 percent protein in terms of calories consumed daily.

🐾 Try to avoid exposure to heavy metals, such as mercury, lead, and cadmium. It's a good idea to test levels of these substances if you have symptoms of hypothyroidism to see if high levels could be exacerbating your symptoms.

🐾 When metabolic and immune function are compromised for an extended time, the damage can show up in the form of conditions such as allergies, digestion problems, and candida overgrowth.

CHAPTER 9

The Importance of Good Adrenal Function

Are you tired? Do you lack energy and find it hard to exercise (or even get up in the morning)? Do you crave sugar? Have you developed mysterious, distressing stomach complaints? Do you find yourself becoming annoyed beyond belief by little things that would have caused no more than a raised eyebrow in years past? A friend once told me that she spent many years with undiagnosed adrenal fatigue, and often felt like she wanted to bite most of the people she talked to. Honestly, at the time I thought she was completely insane until I went through adrenal exhaustion myself, and then the vision of her teeth locked onto to someone's arm started to make more sense.

Your adrenal glands are critical to your health and well-being at any age, but they become even more essential as your hormone levels start to decline with age or illness. Not only are they important in managing all the stress you're bombarded with in your daily life, they also become the major source of sex hormones when ovarian production of these hormones declines during perimenopause and menopause. Given this ovarian connection, it isn't surprising that more women than men end up with adrenal fatigue.

Adrenal problems range widely in severity, from a mild condition that can cause confusing and distressing symptoms to an extreme and sometimes fatal condition known as Addison's disease. Because adrenal hormones impact a broad spectrum of physical, emotional, and psychological functions, from energy and sex drive to the tendency to gain weight, even a mild deficiency can have a profound impact.

HOW DO YOUR ADRENALS AFFECT YOUR THYROID?

Just as your adrenal and ovarian functions are inextricably intertwined, good thyroid function is also necessary for your adrenal glands to function well—and vice versa. The bottom line is hypothyroidism causes stress to your body. And as discussed in chapter 2, stress causes your adrenals to go into overdrive and produce high levels of adrenal hormones, especially cortisol and adrenaline. When stress is ongoing, chronic production of these hormones exhausts your adrenal glands. Unfortunately, this is only the tip of the iceberg. Several other problems occur when adrenal function drops: Without adequate cortisol, T4 can't be converted into active T3, and any T3 you do make, can't be bound by T3 receptors and taken into your cells. In fact, the receptors themselves can become defunct or even disappear in the absence of good adrenal function. You can see how vicious this cycle can become. Low thyroid function leads to excessive adrenal activity, ultimately exhausting the adrenals and compromising adrenal function, which leads to even lower thyroid function. In fact, it's exhausting to even think about!

ADRENAL HORMONES

There are two parts to your adrenal glands. Their inner area, called the *medulla*, produces adrenaline (epinephrine) and noradrenaline (norepinephrine). Their outer area, the *cortex*, produces hormones such as cortisol, aldosterone, and DHEA.

Adrenaline and Noradrenaline

Adrenaline and noradrenaline are our *fight-or-flight* hormones, a name that reflects the purpose they serve: responding to danger. They're also produced when we face sudden or extreme stress or experience even everyday things that cause a surge of strong emotion, such as fear or anger. These hormones increase our heart rate, blood pressure, and blood sugar levels.

Cortisol

Cortisol falls into the class of hormones known as glucocorticoids, which simply means a hormone that affects the metabolism of carbohydrates and, to a lesser extent, fats and proteins. Our bodies produce it continuously, but its levels are highest in the morning and are also elevated by illness or stress.

Cortisol is critical in controlling inflammation and immune response and helps your body recover from all manner of stressors. It affects your chances of developing diseases in the first place and then determines your ability to respond to any chronic illnesses you do develop. It also affects the distribution of stored fat (especially around your waist and at the sides of your face), with excessive levels resulting in an ever-expanding waistline and a rounder face. An exaggerated example is the "moon face" caused by continuous usage of such powerful cortisol drugs as prednisone. On the other hand, once you get to the adrenal burnout stage, you may get thinner, most noticeably in your face. This is why hypothyroidism coupled with very low adrenal function may not result in the weight gain normally associated with low thyroid function. Other important functions of cortisol are regulating cardiovascular and gastrointestinal function and helping control blood sugar. As a result, low adrenal function leads to food cravings and hypoglycemia (low blood sugar).

Aldosterone

Aldosterone is the most important adrenal hormone in the class of hormones called mineralo-corticoids. These hormones help regulate levels of sodium and potassium to control blood pressure, distribution of fluids in the body, and the balance of electrolytes in the blood.

DHEA

DHEA (dehydroepiandrosterone), also made in your adrenal glands, is an androgen, like testosterone. Androgens, a group of hormones that promote the development and maintenance of male secondary sex characteristics, are also produced in smaller quantities in women. They're important in building muscle mass and bone, and have a significant effect on libido, mood, and energy.

DHEA also has many important functions similar to those of cortisol. It has potent anti-inflammatory properties, and people of all ages with chronic inflammatory disease have lower levels of DHEA. It also supports immune function and helps you withstand bacterial and viral diseases (Jiang et al. 1998). DHEA production starts to decline in your late twenties, and declines even further if adrenal function is low.

WHAT HAPPENS WHEN YOUR ADRENALS MALFUNCTION

When you're faced with stressors, your adrenals initially go into overdrive and start to produce increased amounts of various hormones that cause a myriad of physiological changes designed to help you survive. Cortisol pours out, causing your breathing rate, heart rate, and blood pressure to increase, thereby providing your body with more oxygen and nutrients to cope with the stressful situation. Other, less critical body functions, like immune function, digestion, hormone production, and tissue repair, slow down since they aren't as critical to survival.

This can go on without harm for many years if the stressors aren't overwhelming or unremitting, or if your diet and lifestyle choices are extremely healthy. Eventually, however, ongoing stress will cause your adrenals to lose function to the point that you won't produce enough adrenal hormones to carry on normal activities. This state is called *adrenal fatigue*.

Not only can you have too much or too little cortisol, you can also have a disrupted production pattern. Cortisol has a distinct daily production pattern that's quite high an hour after waking and then drops quickly as shown in the chart below. If you don't produce the early morning peak, you may have a hard time getting started in the morning. Or you may have high early morning production but then your levels drop too quickly, leaving you exhausted in the early afternoon. You could also have a reversed pattern: cortisol levels that are low in the morning, increase throughout the day, and peak in the afternoon or evening. This can cause you to have little energy during day and then start to feel better in the late afternoon and feel best after dinner and into the evening. This can potentially result in not being able to fall asleep at a reasonable hour.

Studies have shown that nighttime cortisol levels for fifty-year-olds are about ten to twelve times higher than those of thirty-year-olds, on average. In yet another vicious cycle, this results in a lack of deep, restful sleep, which pushes levels of cortisol even higher (Laughlin and Barret-Connor 2000). These disrupted patterns also result in weight gain, higher levels of glucose and insulin (increasing the risk of diabetes), and higher levels of cholesterol and blood pressure (resulting in heart problems).

Cortisol production pattern

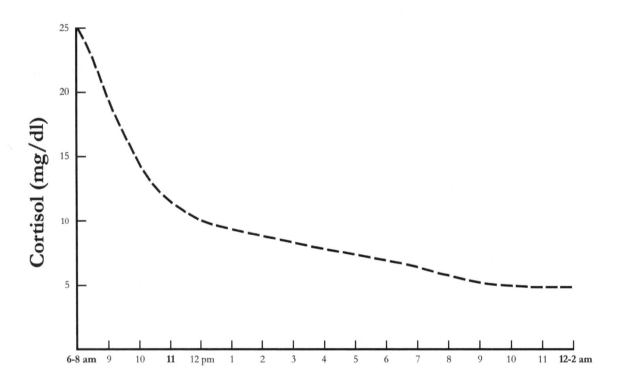

Source: Kathryn Simpson and Dale Bredesen, *The Perimenopause and Menopause Workbook* (Oakland, CA: New Harbinger Publications, 2006).

More Isn't Always Better

Several different problems can occur when your adrenal glands go into overdrive. High cortisol levels coupled with high DHEA levels tell you that your body is experiencing too much stress, either physical or emotional, and your adrenals have increased their hormone output to try to manage the situation. Symptoms of excess cortisol include weight gain (particularly around your middle), stretch marks, irregular periods, bruising, loss of muscle, trouble sleeping, emotional problems such as depression, and excessive hair growth (unfortunately, not where we want it—on our head—but in places like our upper lip and chin). If the situation isn't corrected, your adrenals will start to tire. At this stage, DHEA levels start to drop and cortisol levels generally remain high. If this happens, talk to your doctor about taking supplemental DHEA, as it can be helpful in suppressing your adrenal function if it's pumping out more cortisol than is healthy for you.

Finally, if stress continues, your cortisol level will drop as well, indicating adrenal fatigue, meaning your adrenals are on their way to exhaustion if you don't take steps to halt the downward slide. Alternatively, although not as common, DHEA may remain high while cortisol drops too low. This signals a potential problem with converting pregnenolone to cortisol. Pregnenolone, a hormone made from cholesterol, is sometimes called the "mother hormone" as it's a precursor, or building block, for many other hormones, including cortisol, aldosterone, progesterone, estrogen, testosterone, and DHEA. According to thyroid specialist Barry Durrant-Peatfield, MD, this type of malfunction, where DHEA is elevated and cortisol is low, can only be corrected by supplementing cortisol (Durrant-Peatfield 2003).

Aldosterone levels can also get too high when your adrenals are stressed and in high gear. Elevated aldosterone causes high blood pressure and low potassium levels, which can lead to muscle

Stress and Gender

Several recent studies have uncovered interesting facts about women, stress, and cortisol levels. One found that women who have outside jobs as well as children at home tend to have elevated cortisol levels in the evening (Luecken et al. 1997). Men, on the other hand, have normal, lower cortisol levels. Is this a surprise to any of us? Who makes the dinner, helps with homework, and does the laundry in the evening after work? (An important fact our husbands should also know is that elevated cortisol levels also decrease libido...and they wonder why we're not in the mood!)

Men and women have very different abilities to recover from stress. In response to stress, men's cortisol levels increase more overall, but once the stressor is removed they return to normal much more quickly than women. Also, women report feeling more stressed than men in the same situations, with working women with children reporting the highest stress levels.

cramps, muscle weakness, and numbness or tingling in your extremities. On the other hand, levels of aldosterone can get low when the adrenals are too tired to produce normal levels. Signs of low aldosterone are a reddish, swollen face and indications of water retention, like swollen hands and feet. You should always measure levels of cortisol, DHEA, and aldosterone together, as you may have excesses of one or more of them.

Too Little Adrenal Function Is Even Worse

The onset of adrenal fatigue is often gradual and insidious, and difficult to diagnose in the early stages. Often the situation becomes obvious when an illness or additional stress precipitates a need for additional cortisol that your tired adrenals just can't meet. At this point, your symptoms will become noticeable and affect your ability to function normally.

The most common symptoms of low adrenal function include irritability, fatigue, weakness, anorexia, weight loss, nausea, joint and abdominal pain, diarrhea (which may alternate with constipation), low blood pressure, electrolyte imbalances, hyperpigmentation (dark coloration of the skin), decreased body hair, psychological problems, loss of sex drive, lack of menstrual bleeding, autoimmune conditions like vitiligo, and a general feeling that something's not right.

The seriousness of adrenal fatigue and the symptoms it causes depends on how much adrenal function you've lost and whether you still have the ability to make enough aldosterone despite decreased cortisol production. When aldosterone deficiency is coupled with cortisol deficiency, you're in danger of having a more serious adrenal crisis, which, if severe, can be life threatening.

Salt... It's Not All Bad

Aldosterone regulates how much sodium your body retains and how much it excretes in urine. Since low aldosterone levels result in less sodium being retained, cutting back on salt can worsen some of the symptoms of low aldosterone. Eating more salt doesn't fix the underlying problem of sodium loss caused by low aldosterone levels, but it does temporarily increase the amount of sodium available to your body. When your aldosterone level is low, adding salt can help. Consider using sea salt, as opposed to regular table salt, as it also contains important trace minerals, which are usually removed from table salt. Minimum recommended daily amounts are 1/4 teaspoon to 1/2 teaspoon in water twice a day for women with normal blood pressure. If you have high blood pressure, be sure to talk to your doctor before you try this, to make sure it won't make your condition worse. If you require significantly more salt than this to resolve your symptoms or if you have very low levels of aldosterone on your blood tests, you should talk to your doctor about supplementing with fludrocortisone (Florinef), a drug that has aldosterone-like effects.

Dropping blood pressure and a craving for salt are signals of diminishing aldosterone levels, which can occur even if you take adequate amounts of supplemental cortisol. Other signs are dehydration, which can cause the skin to "tent" when pinched and cause sharp wrinkles to develop, and also make your face and eyes appear sunken. If you have low adrenal function but relatively normal aldosterone production, severe adrenal crisis is rare.

Low levels of DHEA also wreak havoc on your body. DHEA helps your body withstand viral and bacterial diseases (Jiang et al. 1998), so it clearly plays a role in immune function. Low DHEA levels have been associated with increased incidence of autoimmune disease. In addition, DHEA supplementation has proven helpful for people with chronic inflammatory diseases (van Vollenhoven, Engleman, and McGuire 1994).

Liz's Story

Liz's problems started when she went through a traumatic divorce at forty-two. She had been married for eighteen years and had two daughters, ages twelve and fourteen. Up until the divorce, she had managed to stay on top of her very busy life, working full time as a manager of a retail store, keeping up the house, and managing her two daughters' school, sports, and dancing classes.

In her late thirties, Liz had noticed that she had started getting much more tired in the afternoons. She was also getting more easily irritated and short-tempered and started to have trouble sleeping. When she was finally able get to sleep, she would toss and turn, waking up frequently during the night. She went to her doctor for help, and he prescribed an antidepressant, saying it would help with both her mood and her sleep issues. She found that her symptoms got somewhat better and she was less irritable, but her sleeping problems didn't improve.

Despite these health problems, Liz was able to function well and keep her job, the house, and the girls' schedules running smoothly until she learned her husband was having an affair with a coworker. She had believed her marriage was fine, so when she found out from a mutual friend that her husband had been involved with another woman for several months, it came as a horrible shock. Even worse, when she confronted him and gave him an ultimatum, he said he had no intention of giving the other woman up and that he would move out that weekend.

Liz felt as if she had been in a horrible accident. She ached all over and couldn't get out of bed for four days. She had a hard time taking a deep breath and felt as if she was on the verge of passing out when she finally did get up. She wasn't able to go to work for a full week, and when she did go back she felt like she was in a fog and couldn't think straight. She had been a thoroughly organized type A person her entire life. Now it was all she could do to get to work and back and pick up food from a fast-food restaurant for the girls on her way home.

Her daughters hovered around, not knowing what to do. After two months, they called their grandmother and told her that she needed to come and help because they couldn't cope anymore. When Liz's mother arrived three days later, she was horrified by Liz's condition and knew something was very wrong as soon as she saw her. Liz was listless, pale, confused, and unfocused. She had dark circles under her eyes, which also looked sunken. She moved much more slowly than she had previously and got dizzy when she stood up too fast. And despite how tired she was, Liz could hardly get any sleep. She had heart palpitations and felt as if she were shaking inside, which made her sleeping problems even worse. After hearing of all these symptoms, her mother insisted that they call Liz's doctor right way and schedule an appointment.

When Liz saw her doctor a week later, he told her that the stress of her husband leaving her had obviously taken a toll and that she should try to get more rest. He also prescribed an antianxiety drug in addition to her antidepressant medication. Liz took the anxiety medication, but in combination with the antidepressants, it made her feel awful. She was still very shaky but also completely detached and unable to think straight. She continued in this zombielike state for another month until her mother put her foot down and said they needed to get to the bottom of what was going wrong; she didn't want to go home until Liz was able to function normally.

They decided to call Liz's ob-gyn, as she was the only other doctor Liz knew. Her ob-gyn specialized in hormones and menopause and had told Liz at her last appointment that they should consider doing baseline hormone tests because hormones might be a factor in her chronic exhaustion. When Liz explained her symptoms, she told her to come in for some testing. During her appointment, Liz's doctor told her that her blood pressure was very low, and of even greater concern was that it got even lower when she went from lying to standing—an indicator of adrenal fatigue. All of her other symptoms indicated very low cortisol levels, and her lab tests confirmed her doctor's suspicions of adrenal dysfunction. She also had a very elevated TSH level, showing she also had hypothyroidism. Liz's doctor prescribed low-dose cortisol drug therapy to support Liz's adrenals and Armour Thyroid for her hypothyroidism.

Liz started taking the supplemental hormones and felt almost immediate relief from her crushing exhaustion. Over the next few weeks, she found her other symptoms slowly resolving until one day a few months later, she realized she was almost back to her old self. At that point, she worked with her doctor to stop taking the medications for anxiety and depression. Understandably, she was still angry at her husband and distressed about the way her marriage ended, but now she found she was much calmer and able to deal with the situation.

ASSESSING YOUR SYMPTOMS OF ADRENAL DYSFUNCTION

Adrenal fatigue causes few symptoms until cortisol levels fall very low. Doctors receive little or no training in assessing and treating adrenal fatigue in medical school, so they generally don't recognize the symptoms when they encounter them. Infrequently, adrenal fatigue is diagnosed based on laboratory test abnormalities discovered during routine physical exams, such as low levels of sodium, low blood sugar, and high levels of potassium and calcium.

The symptoms of adrenal fatigue are fatigue, dehydration, low blood pressure on standing, low blood sugar, and depression or other emotional problems. Over time, other symptoms appear, such as weight loss, particularly on the sides of the face, and increased skin pigmentation, usually around the nipples and genitals, in the creases of the palms, and on scar tissue). Other symptoms that show up later include bowel problems, such as irritable bowel syndrome, and decreased underarm and genital hair because of the low androgen levels associated with adrenal fatigue.

Along with too much stress for too long, another common cause of adrenal fatigue is hypothyroidism. Autoimmune disease also accounts for many cases of adrenal insufficiency, with thyroid antibodies and thyroid disease also found in some cases (Blizzard, Chee, and Davis 1967).

Looking at symptoms is important in getting to the bottom of your adrenal status. In fact, it's just as critical as measuring levels of specific adrenal hormones. The following evaluation will help you assess your symptoms so you can determine whether adrenal fatigue may be a factor for you.

EXERCISE: Adrenal Fatigue Symptom Evaluation

In this evaluation, you may notice that several symptoms of adrenal fatigue are similar to those of hypothyroidism. In truth, these two conditions are so closely intertwined that it's often hard to tell them apart. Read the statements below, decide on the level of severity or frequency of each sign or symptom, and then circle the number that most accurately reflects how that statement applies to you:

0 = None or never   1 = Mild or occasionally

2 = Moderate or often   3 = Severe or always

At the bottom of each page, total up the points circled, then carry these totals forward to the end of the evaluation to get a final score.

0	1	2	3	I have symptoms of low thyroid function. I tried thyroid hormone supplementation and felt better for a little while, and then I felt worse.
0	1	2	3	I have a pale face and lips.
0	1	2	3	I have panic attacks or anxiety.
0	1	2	3	I have eczema or psoriasis.
0	1	2	3	I get neck, back, or groin pain.
0	1	2	3	I'm sensitive to heat and cold.

Page total: _____

0	1	2	3	My cheeks or eyes appear sunken.
0	1	2	3	I have dark circles under my eyes.
0	1	2	3	I'm tired a lot of the time.
0	1	2	3	I feel better when I'm lying down.
0	1	2	3	I get cold sweats.
0	1	2	3	I have bowel problems.
0	1	2	3	I crave sweets.
0	1	2	3	I can't seem to stop drinking alcohol.
0	1	2	3	Sometimes I feel like I'm going to faint.
0	1	2	3	I feel like I'm shaking or shivering inside.
0	1	2	3	I'm irritable and moody.
0	1	2	3	Simple things have become confusing and even overwhelming for me.
0	1	2	3	I've developed allergies.
0	1	2	3	I have a hard time getting going in the morning.
0	1	2	3	I crave salty food.
0	1	2	3	I have environmental sensitivities. Scents like perfume, chemicals, or air pollution bother me.
0	1	2	3	I have a lot of respiratory or sinus infections that sometimes last for several weeks.
0	1	2	3	I have thin, dry skin.
0	1	2	3	I can't handle stress, and I feel ill or shaken after stressful events.
0	1	2	3	I drive myself constantly and feel like I can never catch up.
0	1	2	3	When I introduce people, I panic and forget their names.
0	1	2	3	I seem to get sick a lot and have a hard time bouncing back.
0	1	2	3	I feel best after dinner.
0	1	2	3	I have to drink coffee or other caffeinated beverages to keep going.
0	1	2	3	I often feel guilty or blame others.

Page total: _____

0	1	2	3	I often feel tired or depressed, but eating sweets makes me feel better.
0	1	2	3	I often have abdominal pain, gas, or an upset stomach.
0	1	2	3	I avoid social engagements.
0	1	2	3	Light bothers my eyes much more than it used to, and I'm uncomfortable when I don't wear sunglasses.
0	1	2	3	Different parts of my body have turned strange colors or the creases of my joints appear darker.
0	1	2	3	Sometimes I can't take deep breaths.
0	1	2	3	When I press on the area of my back at the bottom of the rib cage near my spine, it hurts.
0	1	2	3	I crave sweets, chocolate, and foods made with white flour.
0	1	2	3	I'm especially sensitive to color, sound, and odor.
0	1	2	3	When I get up quickly from a reclining position, I get dizzy or everything gets dim. Sometimes I even black out.
0	1	2	3	I get angry easily and start yelling. It takes me a long time to recover.
0	1	2	3	I can't concentrate and my memory isn't good.
0	1	2	3	I have signs of dehydration, such as sharp wrinkles, and my skin forms stiff folds when pinched.
0	1	2	3	I have difficulty processing information and feel like I'm not as smart as I used to be.
0	1	2	3	I feel isolated and don't want to talk to people or do any of the things I used to.
0	1	2	3	I have inflammatory bowel disease or irritable bowel syndrome.
0	1	2	3	I have insomnia.
0	1	2	3	I smoke cigarettes.
0	1	2	3	I have low blood pressure or a weak or slow pulse.
0	1	2	3	I'm losing body hair.
0	1	2	3	I'm losing weight for no reason and my face has gotten thin.
0	1	2	3	I have a hard time exercising because I get tired easily.
0	1	2	3	I get heart palpitations.

Page total: _____

0	1	2	3	Sometimes I wake up at night and have a hard time breathing.
0	1	2	3	I get hissing sounds in my ears.
0	1	2	3	I have an autoimmune disease.
0	1	2	3	I get fainting spells.
0	1	2	3	I have asthma.
0	1	2	3	My muscles are weak and stiff.

Page total: _____

Total number of points: _____

Interpreting Your Results

If your total points are between 15 and 20 (or if you have several of these symptoms or one particularly bothersome one, such as irritable bowel syndrome), you may be beginning to show signs of low adrenal function. A score between 21 and 26 indicates the deficiency is more serious, and a score over 26 indicates that significant adrenal deficiency is likely (with probable thyroid involvement). With any of these results, have a complete physical, including lab tests to measure blood or saliva levels of cortisol and DHEA and blood levels of aldosterone and ACTH (adrenocorticotropic hormone, the pituitary hormone that stimulates production of cortisol). Since your adrenals are affected by your other endocrine glands, it's also important to measure levels of free T3, free T4, TSH, and reverse T3, as well as thyroid antibodies if your doctor feels it's warranted. (See chapter 6 for more on these tests.) Because of the interrelationship between all of the endocrine glands, it's also important to measure levels of FSH, estrogen, progesterone, and testosterone.

TESTING YOUR ADRENAL FUNCTION

The symptoms in the preceding evaluation all suggest low adrenal function. However, some of them may have other causes, particularly low levels of estrogen or thyroid hormones, so lab tests are necessary to determine the exact status of your adrenal function. I'll describe the relevant lab tests in detail, but first let's take a quick look at some simple tests you can do at home to help you get some idea if you might have adrenal fatigue.

Tests You Can Do at Home

There are three simple tests you can do at home to determine whether you may have adrenal fatigue: the pupil contraction test, a blood pressure test, and the white line test. If any of these tests indicate possible adrenal dysfunction, make an appointment with your doctor to have your adrenal function evaluated.

PUPIL CONTRACTION TEST

In the early 1900s, it was discovered that the pupil is a very accurate indicator of low adrenal function as its ability to contract and stay contracted when exposed to light is controlled in large part by your adrenals. If your adrenals are fatigued, your pupil won't be able to remain contracted and will dilate unnaturally. To do this test you'll need a mirror, a flashlight, and a watch.

In a darkened room with a mirror on the wall (a bathroom is a good choice), look into the mirror and then hold the flashlight at the side of your head with the light pointing toward your temple. Shine the light across the front of your eyes and observe how your pupil reacts.

Your pupil should contract and stay contracted as the light hits it. If, after a short period of time (two minutes or less), it starts to dilate, then contracts, then dilates, and doesn't stay contracted, you most likely have some level of adrenal fatigue. Mild fatigue may not show up with this test.

BLOOD PRESSURE TEST

Adrenal fatigue is one of the primary causes of low blood pressure, or hypotension. If your blood pressure drops when you rise from lying down to standing up (the opposite of what normally happens), you may have low adrenal function. You will need a blood pressure monitor to do this test.

Lie down and relax for five to ten minutes, then take your blood pressure while still lying flat. Next, stand up and take your blood pressure again. When you stand, your blood pressure should go up about 10 mm Hg. If it drops instead, you may have adrenal fatigue.

WHITE LINE TEST

This test was developed in 1917 by a French doctor, Emile Sergent. It isn't the most accurate indicator, as only about 40 percent of people with low adrenal function test positive, but if you do test positive, it's almost certain that you have low adrenal function. All you need to do this test is a ballpoint pen.

Using the dull end of the pen, make a mark about six inches long across your abdomen (don't press overly hard or scratch the skin). If your adrenals are fatigued, the line will widen and stay white for about two minutes.

Lab Tests for Adrenal Function

If you have several of the symptoms of adrenal fatigue listed in the evaluation, particularly severe fatigue, it's important to test your levels of the key adrenal hormones: cortisol, aldosterone, DHEA (in the sulfate form), and ACTH. Cortisol and aldosterone should be tested in the first week of your menstrual cycle. (If you're postmenopausal, anytime is fine.) Because they're made from progesterone, the higher progesterone levels that occur midcycle can raise levels of cortisol and aldosterone. To accurately assess adrenal function, it's important to gauge your lowest levels.

CORTISOL TESTS

The most widely accepted test for cortisol is a blood test. Since you need to test cortisol more than once a day to determine your production pattern, you will need to go to the lab at least twice in one day to have blood drawn. Most doctors suggest 8 a.m. and 4 p.m.

Saliva testing is more convenient, as samples can be collected anywhere, even at work. Plus, this allows you to test at four different times during the day, giving you a more accurate picture of your production pattern. Most doctors recommend measuring levels at 8 a.m., 12 noon, 4 p.m., and 10 p.m. (or six times, adding midnight and 4 a.m., if you're game). According to Dr. Michael Borkin, director of research at Sabre Sciences (personal communications), "Salivary tests are extremely valuable in assessing adrenal function, as the elevations or decreases in cortisol levels at different points during the day will reflect where the stress is originating. These fluctuations in levels are extremely important even if levels are within normal ranges. The cortisol level at 8 a.m. gives insight into the size and status of your adrenal glands: If your adrenals are enlarged, indicting they are in overdrive, you will have high cortisol levels; and if they are atrophied or shrinking, you are on your way to adrenal fatigue and your levels will be low."

Dr. Borkin also says that a drop from 8 a.m. to noon can indicate an inflammatory process. A drop of 50 percent or more is usually associated with problems with the digestive system, while a drop in excess of 70 percent usually indicates a parasitic infestation. The noon measurement is especially reflective of blood sugar control, and levels at 4 p.m. give insight into chronic infections, with elevated levels generally indicating bacterial overgrowth and low levels indicating viral infections. Cortisol levels at 8 p.m. are associated with your ability to utilize insulin and can indicate insulin resistance or type 2 diabetes. The midnight measurement is important because elevated cortisol at this time can interfere with the release of growth hormone and proper immune function. Spiking at 4 a.m., which is abnormal, shows your blood sugar reserves have run out, so your adrenals have increased their output of cortisol to bring your blood sugar back into normal range.

The twenty-four-hour urine test is also valuable, as it reveals exactly how much cortisol you produce over a twenty-four-hour period. However, it won't detect a disrupted pattern, and it needs to be done on a day when you can stay close to the collection container all day. Your doctor will most likely have a preference for one type of testing methodology.

ALDOSTERONE TESTS

Testing for aldosterone may be done by either a twenty-four-hour urine test or a blood test. You should avoid salting your food for twenty-four hours before the test. For a complete picture, talk to your doctor about testing levels of sodium and potassium as well as renin, an enzyme released by the kidneys to stimulate production of aldosterone by the adrenals. Renin levels go up when aldosterone is low.

ACTH TESTS

ACTH, a hormone produced by the pituitary, stimulates your adrenals to produce cortisol. Testing ACTH levels will determine whether low cortisol production is caused by pituitary dysfunction or by a problem with your adrenals themselves, just like levels of TSH, also produced by the pituitary, can be helpful in assessing the root cause of low levels of thyroid hormones. Low ACTH coupled with low cortisol levels signals a problem with your pituitary because it should have detected low levels of cortisol and increased levels of ACTH to stimulate additional production. High levels of ACTH coupled with low levels of cortisol signals a problem with your adrenal glands, as they aren't responding to the command from your pituitary to produce more cortisol. Your doctor may want to wait to see if your cortisol level is low before measuring ACTH. This is done by a blood test anytime during your menstrual cycle.

If abnormalities are found in your cortisol or ACTH tests, your doctor may want to do an ACTH stimulation test. This test assesses adrenal reserves and is an indicator of adrenal fatigue. First baseline cortisol levels are tested, then ACTH is injected. Cortisol is measured again after thirty and sixty minutes to see how your adrenals responded. If they're functioning properly, your cortisol level should double.

DHEA SULFATE (DHEA-S) TEST

It's important to measure the sulfate form of DHEA, as this is the principal adrenal hormone, other than cortisol, secreted in response to ACTH. Low levels of DHEA sulfate indicate low adrenal function. Testing should be done first thing in the morning.

TREATING ADRENAL FATIGUE

Problems involving either overstimulation or fatigue of the adrenal glands are generally overlooked in conventional medicine. Although the importance of the adrenals for overall health has been recognized for over a century, it's unlikely that your doctor will consider them when evaluating your thyroid health, or your health in general. Even endocrinologists, who specialize in hormone health, focus primarily on extreme, life-threatening conditions such as Addison's disease (drastically low adrenal function) and Cushing's disease (drastically overactive adrenals).

This unfortunate situation makes it essential that you educate yourself about adrenal function. You should analyze your symptoms carefully and be prepared to explain anything you find to your doctor. You may have to make a case for taking the next step: measuring your levels of adrenal hormones. This effort is well worth it, as your adrenal glands have the miraculous capacity to regain full functionality if given the right support. Low dosages of bioidentical cortisol, and aldosterone supplementation if necessary, can give fatigued adrenals a much-needed rest. If your symptoms and test results show deficiencies of these key hormones, you should explore the following treatment options with your doctor.

Supplemental Cortisol

People with adrenal fatigue indicated by low cortisol levels on blood tests may be treated with hydrocortisone (Cortef), which is simply bioidentical cortisol. The daily replacement dose for most women is 10 to 25 mg, which can be taken in two to four divided doses. Some doctors recommend mimicking the body's normal production pattern by taking a large dose first thing in the morning, a smaller dose four hours later, and then even smaller doses four and eight hours later. The body naturally makes around 35 to 40 mg per day, so even 25 mg won't shut your body's production of cortisol down, although it will reduce your body's production slightly. The supplemental cortisol will replenish your adrenal reserves and return them to normal, healthy levels. Most doctors recommend using cortisol replacement for two to four months and then tapering off and retesting to see if you've regained your adrenal function. You may only need to take cortisol for a short time, or it may take one to two years to regain function if your fatigue is severe.

During illness or surgery, doctors generally recommend increasing doses up to two to three times the usual level for three days. During major illness or surgery, or in the case of an accident, high doses of five or more times the normal dose may be required to avoid an adrenal crisis.

The alternative to bioidentical cortisol is a longer-acting synthetic form of cortisol such as prednisone (Deltasone) and prednisolone (Prelone). These drugs have more long-lasting effects on the body and dangerous side effects, such as loss of lean body mass and bone density and increased visceral fat. Nevertheless, many doctors prefer to use these drugs because they're more familiar with them, and unfortunately, they often don't understand the difference between natural, bioidentical cortisol and chemically altered forms (Jefferies 1996). It's worth it to try to find a doctor who's open to considering this gentler, more natural alternative to rebuilding adrenal function.

Supplemental Aldosterone

Low aldosterone is generally treated with fludrocortisone (Florinef), a form of aldosterone. Most doctors prescribe a daily dose of 100 mcg. Because starting at this level can cause side effects, doctors generally recommend starting with one-fourth of a pill (25 mcg) and raising the dose by 25 mcg every five to seven days until you get to 100 mcg. The effects should be noticed in two to four weeks with this approach, or in one week if you start at 100 mcg. You may also get bioidentical aldosterone by prescription at a compounding pharmacy (see the Resources section).

Supplemental DHEA

Oral DHEA can be purchased over the counter, without a prescription. The dose most doctors recommend for women is 15 mg (unless you're being treated for rheumatoid arthritis, in which case 50 to 100 mg is recommended). DHEA can effectively block estrogen, so if your estrogen levels are low, you should start at a low dose and work up. Because the body can convert DHEA to testosterone, if you have a high testosterone level you should also be careful using DHEA and start low. Symptoms of excessive DHEA include acne, sugar cravings, weight gain, fatigue, anger, depression, insomnia, restless sleep, mood swings, irritability, and, for women, excess facial hair and deepening of the voice. When supplementing DHEA, you should work closely with your doctor to monitor blood levels and symptoms.

Adrenal Extracts

Supplements made from bovine adrenal glands may also help rebuild your adrenal glands. Glandular products contain many substances, including hormones, but it's hard to quantify the levels of hormones in these products, since they can vary from animal to animal and from batch to batch. A product often recommended by doctors specializing in this field is Isocort, made by the German company Bezwecken. You can purchase adrenal extracts at most natural food stores or online.

Other Ways to Support Your Adrenal Function

As with thyroid function, lifestyle choices can have a profound impact on adrenal function. One obvious way to support your adrenals is by taking whatever steps you can to reduce stress in your life. But since some stress is inevitable, it's also worthwhile to develop stress management skills. Even something as simple as breathing deeply can have a profound impact on how your body responds to stress. There are many excellent books and other resources on stress management. Check out a few so you can find an approach that works for you.

On a physical level, all of the recommendations in chapter 8 will be helpful. In addition, here are a few specific recommendations for adrenal health in regard to exercise, food choices, and supplements.

THE BENEFITS OF EXERCISE

One of the best antidotes to high cortisol levels is regular exercise, as it reduces excess cortisol production. Research suggests that it doesn't take much exercise to be beneficial. As little as thirty minutes of exercise a day, three to five days a week, can have an effect (Mayo Foundation for Medical Education and Research 2007). But be careful not to overdo it, since too much extremely taxing exercise can have the opposite effect and cause testosterone levels to decline and cortisol levels to rise. When beginning an exercise program or increasing your activity level, it's a good idea to work your way up slowly. As you have more energy and stamina, you can exercise more vigorously.

DIET

Consuming foods you're allergic to or don't tolerate well can take a toll on your adrenal glands over time. If you suspect you have food allergies, you should talk to your doctor about having allergy testing done. An optimal, balanced diet, as described in chapter 8, will help support your adrenal function—and the rest of your body too!

In terms of controlling cortisol levels, it's important to avoid eating excessive amounts of simple carbohydrates (sugar, white flour products, and other refined grains). These foods elevate both blood sugar levels and insulin production, signaling the adrenals to release cortisol. This creates a vicious cycle, as elevated cortisol levels cause the pancreas to secrete even more insulin. If this continues long enough, it can ultimately lead to diabetes.

There are several basic rules to follow that help normalize levels of blood sugar, insulin and cortisol: Don't skip meals. This causes the adrenals to release cortisol. Instead, eat at regular intervals throughout the day and try to include complex carbohydrates, protein, and good-quality fats at every meal. Avoid stimulants such as energy drinks that contain caffeine and ephedra-like compounds. If you do drink caffeine, try to avoid it after noon.

Certain nutrients support the adrenals: the B vitamins (especially vitamin B_5, or pantothenic acid), vitamin C, magnesium, and zinc. You can take these in the form of supplements, or you can try to include more food sources of these nutrients in your diet. Here are some good food sources of each (Haas and Levin 2006):

- **B vitamins:** nutritional yeast, whole grains, and some beans, peas, and nuts (nutritional yeast being the only good vegetarian source of B_{12})

- **Vitamin B_5:** widely available, with good sources including egg yolks, fish, chicken, whole grains, peanuts, dried beans, and many vegetables

- **Vitamin C:** most fruits and vegetables, especially citrus fruits, papaya, cantaloupe, strawberries, bell peppers, broccoli, tomatoes, and dark leafy greens

- **Magnesium:** dark leafy greens, whole grains, and most nuts, seeds, and legumes

- **Zinc:** most meats, seafoods, and poultry and, to a lesser extent, whole grains, nuts, and seeds

HELPFUL SUPPLEMENTS

A variety of herbs are effective at reducing elevated cortisol levels, especially phosphatidylserine and ashwagandha. Phosphatidylserine is believed to repair cortisol receptors in the hypothalamus that are damaged by high cortisol levels. This damage reduces the hypothalamus's ability to detect and correct ongoing high levels of cortisol levels. Phosphatidylserine also helps repair the feedback control function that normally corrects both high and low cortisol levels. Typical dosages are one to three 100 mg capsules per day. Ashwagandha helps reduce levels of cortisol. The typical dose is 250 mg per day. Pregnenolone, discussed earlier in this chapter, can also normalize cortisol levels, bringing them down if they're high and raising them if they're low. Your dose should be decided on after testing blood levels, but it's usually between 10 and 50 mg per day. It can be purchased over the counter at many natural food stores or online.

WHAT'S NEXT?

Now that you've completed the Adrenal Fatigue Symptom Evaluation, you should have a much better understanding of your adrenal status. If your responses indicate low adrenal function, schedule an appointment with your doctor as soon as possible so that you can have your adrenal function evaluated. Take a copy of the completed evaluation with you to your appointment to give your doctor a complete picture of your symptoms. Remember, it's always important to evaluate your adrenal function when you evaluate your thyroid function—initially as well as periodically during thyroid treatment.

At this point in the book, you probably have a good idea of your own thyroid health, your symptoms, and the cause of any dysfunction. Hopefully you've found a good doctor, had lab tests of hormone levels, and started on a treatment program—one that includes any needed changes in your lifestyle. If you have children, it's also important to assess their thyroid function. In addition to sharing your genes, your children probably share many elements of your lifestyle and environment. This combination of factors puts them at heightened risk for thyroid dysfunction as well. The next chapter is devoted to helping you assess their thyroid health. Then, chapter 11 will discuss hyperthyroidism.

KEY POINTS

🖎 The adrenals make many important hormones that help your body manage stress, including cortisol and DHEA. In addition, your adrenal glands become the major source of sex hormones when production of these hormones hormone declines during perimenopause.

🖎 Good thyroid function is necessary for your adrenal glands to function well. Both the amount of cortisol you make and your body's ability to utilize it are affected when you have low thyroid function. Supplementing thyroid hormones can place added demands on your adrenals and contribute to adrenal fatigue, so if you take thyroid medication it's important to also assess your adrenal function and treat any deficiencies.

🖎 Cortisol keeps your body's reactions to stress in balance and prevents stress from harming your body. It also helps regulate cardiovascular and gastrointestinal function and helps control blood sugar, so low adrenal function can lead to food cravings and hypoglycemia.

🖎 Either too much or too little cortisol is bad for you, and your daily pattern of cortisol production is also important. Symptoms of excess cortisol include weight gain (particularly around your middle), stretch marks, irregular periods, bruising, excessive hair growth, loss of muscle, trouble sleeping and emotional problems such as depression.

🖎 Adrenal fatigue can be caused by many different things, including ongoing excessive cortisol production, low thyroid function, and autoimmune disease, and can result in a large number of symptoms.

🖎 If your symptom evaluation indicates you may have adrenal dysfunction, schedule an appointment with your doctor to assess your adrenal function and have the needed lab tests done. Your doctor should test levels of cortisol, aldosterone, ACTH, and DHEA sulfate. While waiting for your doctor's appointment, you can also try the simple home tests described in this chapter.

🖎 Supplemental cortisol can help rebuild your adrenal function. Supplemental aldosterone or DHEA may also be helpful.

🖎 To effectively treat adrenal dysfunction, it's important to reduce or manage your stress. In addition, exercise, a nutritious diet, and certain supplements can all help support your adrenal health.

CHAPTER 10

Signs of Thyroid Dysfunction in Children

There is nothing more important than our kids' health. When they suffer, we suffer. It's distressing enough when we start to lose thyroid function at middle age, but the effects of low thyroid function on your children can be devastating—and can compromise their health for life. If you or other family members have hypothyroidism or another type of thyroid disease, it's likely that your children do too. It's worth having them tested to see if this is the case, as it's never too soon to treat hypothyroidism in children.

Hypothyroidism occurs at all ages—even in infants. In centuries past, *cretinism*, a serious condition that results in severe retardation, occurred when babies were born without the ability to produce adequate thyroid hormones, which are critical for development of the brain and body before and after birth. Fortunately, this is much less common today, as thyroid hormone testing has become a standard part of the tests all children undergo at birth in the United States. However, even mild hypothyroidism in either the mother or the baby can result in varying degrees of abnormal physical and mental development.

If we don't detect low thyroid function in children and stop it in its tracks, the outcome is bleak: Through no fault of their own, kids with thyroid dysfunction can be labeled "problem" children. And they grow into adults who are labeled "hysterical" or "hypochondriacal" because of chronic, vague symptoms of fatigue, irritability, headaches, intestinal disorders, pain, and other ailments that may seem mysterious but are actually indications of low thyroid function. A simple symptom evaluation followed by a blood test of thyroid hormone levels can detect thyroid problems early and profoundly change the course of your child's life.

GESTATION

Even as a fetus, a child can be affected by inadequate thyroid function. A baby has two sources of thyroid hormones: its own thyroid and its mother's. The mother transfers enough thyroid hormones across the placenta to meet her baby's needs for about the first ten to twelve weeks of gestation. After that point, the fetus develops the ability to synthesize its own thyroid hormones.

Because thyroid hormones play such a critical role in growth and development, low thyroid function can be devastating at any point in the process. Even a slight deficiency can result in low birth weight, lifelong small stature, and developmental abnormalities. There are three basic thyroid conditions that can impact a baby's development during pregnancy:

- Hypothyroidism in the mother is a serious risk factor for the baby and can result in a multitude of developmental problems. Clinical studies have shown that even mild maternal hypothyroidism can lead to developmental deficiencies in children, causing learning difficulties and slightly lower performance on IQ tests (Haddow et al. 1999). The most common cause of subclinical hypothyroidism in the mother is autoimmune disease, in which case thyroid antibodies can cross the placenta and attack the baby's thyroid gland, compromising its ability to function, as well.

- Insufficient function of the baby's thyroid gland or pituitary gland (which regulates the thyroid) can also result in inadequate production of thyroid hormones and impact the baby's development. Most babies with this condition are normal at birth because their mother's thyroid hormones provide enough thyroid support during gestation. But if it isn't detected and treated immediately after birth, mental and developmental disabilities develop rapidly.

- Iodine deficiency is the most common preventable thyroid-related cause of developmental problems, including mental retardation, in the world. Inadequate iodine intake causes hypothyroidism in both mother and fetus. If this deficiency isn't corrected during the first or second trimester, the child can develop mental retardation, deaf-mutism, and spasticity (stiff, rigid muscles or involuntary muscle spasms). Treatment during the third trimester or after birth will not prevent these birth defects.

Warning signs indicating maternal hypothyroidism include premature birth of an underweight baby or a long gestation period of a baby weighing more than nine pounds (Waller et al. 2000). If you experienced either of these situations, you should be on the alert for other symptoms of low thyroid function in both you and your children.

INFANCY

Obvious signs of hypothyroidism at birth other than low or high birth weight are jaundice (causing a yellowing of the baby's skin), an umbilical hernia (an abnormal bulge or protrusion that can be seen or felt over the belly button), or edema (LaFranchi et al. 1979). However, relatively mild thyroid deficiency may not be readily apparent in newborns. Other signs to look for include being quieter and more lethargic than other babies or needing more sleep. Their breathing may be somewhat noisy, which makes them appear to have a cold much of the time, and they also tend to breath through their mouths due to swollen nasal passages. Their cries are often hoarse or softer than normal.

Physically, their lips and the area around their eyes may be swollen and their hair may be straight and coarse. Their faces may be broader than normal and lack expression, resulting in a somewhat apathetic appearance. This dull appearance is compounded by the baby's inability to shut its mouth due to breathing difficulties or a swollen, protruding tongue. A sign of significant hypothyroidism is a depressed or flattened bridge of the nose, sometimes called a saddle nose. Infants with hypothyroidism may have eyes that are more deeply set than usual and larger than normal heads, which are seemingly hard to support and tend to fall forward. This is a result of the seams of tissue that connect the bones in the head hardening and closing more slowly than usual. The abdomen often protrudes more than normal, sometimes due to constipation, and these children may fail to gain weight at a normal rate.

These babies are often less active than other children their age, both physically and mentally. They fail to notice objects around them and appear to lack curiosity. Content to lie still for long periods of time, they aren't inclined to attempt to sit up, creep, crawl, stand, or walk, and they often lack the muscular coordination to do so. Although it is more common for these children to be listless, some are the opposite: very nervous and prone to scream and cry at the least provocation. Low thyroid function also results in many of the physical characteristics seen in adults, especially weight gain that causes a fat, flabby appearance.

Development of teeth can be delayed, and the teeth may be malformed or misplaced, with crowding or gaps and numerous cavities. Enamel can be defective, so teeth grind down more quickly and their crowns are poorly faceted. These irregularities are common in both baby teeth and permanent teeth.

These symptoms are a signal to talk to your pediatrician about evaluating your baby's thyroid function. It is critical to detect and treat low thyroid function as early as possible. A very small amount of supplemental thyroid hormones can work miracles for these infants and allow them to develop normally and reach their full potential.

EARLY CHILDHOOD

When thyroid deficiency continues untreated into childhood, it results in continued decline in mental and physical development, and often behavior problems. Many of these children are quieter and slower than others, sleep longer than other children of the same age, and have a hard time getting started in the morning. But paradoxically, some become hyperactive and are nervous, overly aggressive, and given to fits of rage. Emotional problems are common. These children may cry for no apparent reason or throw temper tantrums. They may also lack self-confidence. They fight rules and restrictions and generally have a short attention span, jumping from one activity to another.

They aren't able to sit quietly and study, which causes problems in school. They also often have problems interacting with other children due to this lack of emotional control.

When you're trying to get to the bottom of what may be going on with your child's thyroid function, it's very important to understand that symptoms are highly individualized and can seem contradictory. It's commonly thought that this is due to the relative severity of the hypothyroid condition, or it may be due to individual biochemical makeup. Just as people react in different ways to medication—some of us get overstimulated by over-the-counter cold medication and some us pass out—individuals react differently to hypothyroidism. The fact that some children are quieter and more subdued and some are hyperactive and out of control clearly demonstrates this dichotomy in individual response to the disease and is also seen in many symptoms covered below, such as growth rate.

Still, there are some common symptoms in childhood hypothyroidism. Bed-wetting past the age of six or seven is a key indicator of low thyroid function and should always be explored. This isn't something a child with hypothyroidism can control, but nonetheless the humiliation associated with this condition is traumatic to the child (and the parents!). Fortunately, it's often easily resolved by supplementation with thyroid hormones.

Children with hypothyroidism tend to have swollen lymph glands and problems with adenoids and their tonsils. The uvula can swell along with the tonsils, causing loud breathing, snoring, and an inability to breath through the mouth. Unsuccessful tonsillectomies and adenoidectomies are also much more common in these children, as their tonsils and adenoids have a tendency to grow back. Treatment with thyroid hormones results in a decrease in the size of these tissues and also prevents them from growing back (Barker, Hoskins, and Mosenthal 1922). These children also have lowered immunity and therefore a heightened susceptibility to infection, leading to more frequent respiratory infections and sore throats.

Thomas's Story

In second grade, Thomas started to have a hard time keeping up in school. His teacher referred him to a school counselor to evaluate him for potential learning disabilities. His tests showed he was of above-average intelligence, but he was having a hard time understanding instructions and processing information. The counselor recommended that Thomas start working with a learning disabilities specialist. The specialist recommended tutoring, as well as Ritalin (methylphenidate) for ADHD. His parents agreed to the tutoring but decided to hold off on starting the Ritalin after reading about the drugs potential side effects.

Thomas had other problems that were troublesome. He was still wetting his bed at age eight. He was also very emotional and had a hard time taking direction from his teacher and his parents. The least little bit of criticism would result in anger or tears. This caused his classmates to make fun of him, and as a result, he had no close friends.

A persistent rash that looked like eczema was the catalyst for a visit to the doctor that changed Thomas's life. His doctor did a full physical, and on hearing of his learning disability and other symptoms, did thyroid tests. Thomas's pediatrician had seen so many cases of ADHD respond to thyroid medication that he suspected low thyroid function right away. The tests proved him right; Thomas's TSH was above the recommended 3.0 mU/l treatment threshold. He started Thomas on a low dose of Armour Thyroid, and Thomas responded to the treatment within the first month. The first thing his parents noticed was that his rash started to resolve, then they realized he had gone for almost two weeks without wetting the bed. After a month or two, his counselor and teacher both remarked on a marked improvement in his schoolwork and his ability to concentrate. Thomas also became much calmer and less emotional. As a result, he started to get along much better with his classmates, and eventually other kids in his class started to invite him over and include him in social activities. After six months, all of his symptoms were resolved.

PUBERTY

Puberty is a time of drastic physical and emotional changes triggered by a complex interplay of hormones. It's characterized by accelerated growth and development, which often cause existing symptoms of thyroid deficiency to become more pronounced. In all stages of childhood, hypothyroidism affects sexual characteristics, physical growth, cognitive function, and emotions, but the hormonal changes of puberty can heighten the effects and cause a myriad of symptoms such as fatigue, diminished endurance, nervous behavior, mood swings, digestive problems, skin problems, weight gain, and constipation. In addition, undiagnosed thyroid problems are often behind recurring illnesses and health problems during puberty.

Many teenage girls suffer from thyroid disorders these days. Instead of bubbling over with the natural exuberance usually seen in girls this age, these girls become quite and reserved or, worse, high-strung and irritable. They burst into tears or angry outbursts at the least provocation, with a diagnosis of "suspected bipolar disorder" becoming almost common. They suffer from symptoms like headaches and usually have constipation, which further compromises their situation as it causes absorption of toxins from their intestines. They tend to have skin problems, with ache and even boils adding to the general misery and making them more withdrawn. Thyroid therapy seems almost miraculous in its ability to restore these young women to normal health and functioning.

Sexual Development

Thyroid hormone levels have a profound effect on sexual development. An obvious sign of low levels in younger girls is swollen genitalia and underdeveloped labia. Further, the breasts and uterus remain undersized. Boy's sexual glands are also often immature and undersized.

Conversely, low thyroid function can also be a cause of precocious puberty, which is a rapidly growing problem in the United States. If the pituitary gland releases hormones that stimulate the gonads to produce sex hormones too early, some children may begin to go through puberty at an excessively young age—even as early as seven or eight. The way this works is that hypothyroidism causes the hypothalamus to increase production of thyrotropin-releasing hormone, which in turn causes the pituitary to increase its production of thyroid-stimulating hormone. This elevates levels of follicle-stimulating hormone and results in premature ovarian production of estrogen and early onset of puberty (Duncan 1998). Supplementing thyroid hormones when precocious puberty begins has been successful in stopping and reversing it and its symptoms, such as breast development and pubic hair growth (Anasti et al. 1995).

On the other hand, milder cases of hypothyroidism may cause everything to slow down and result in the child reaching puberty at a later age. Low thyroid hormone levels can cause other problems related to sexual development, too. For girls, this generally shows up as problems with menstrual cycles, such as heavy bleeding that may cause low-grade anemia, further depleting their already low energy stores. Other common symptoms include severe menstrual cramps, exaggerated PMS symptoms, and irregular periods.

Physical Growth

Thyroid hormones play an important role in the development of the brain and nervous system in children and teenagers. Adequate thyroid function is necessary for bone growth and the development of strong bones, so timing of treatment is extremely important to your child's future. Treatment must begin before the growth plates in the bones close if the child is to achieve normal size and growth. This is generally before the age of twenty, although some cases of additional growth up to age thirty have been reported. It's common for rapid growth to occur after thyroid supplementation begins—even up to four to five inches very quickly—which then subsides and follows a natural growth curve.

Although childhood growth may be stunted by extreme hypothyroidism, a minor deficiency of thyroid hormones at puberty can actually interfere with growth in such a way that the adolescent becomes unusually tall instead. Thyroid hormones play a part in causing growth plates at the end of each long bone to close normally. A deficiency can prevent this from happening, allowing growth to continue for a longer period of time than normal, causing greater than normal height. Another physical anomaly found in girls with hypothyroidism is a pelvis that's smaller than normal and narrow hips.

Hypothyroidism also affects muscle function and ligaments, which are crucial for support of the bones and for the overall structure and function of the body. When muscles and ligaments are looser and more flexible than they should be in growing children, it can result in conditions such as scoliosis, knock-knees, flat feet, chronic sprains, and kneecaps given to dislocation.

The Brain and Cognition

The brain, with its high concentration of T3 thyroid receptors, must have adequate amounts of this hormone to work properly and to understand and process information. Children who are deficient in thyroid hormones have a progressively harder time coping with the demands of school as classes get harder at higher grade levels. Hypothyroidism has also been linked with reduced overall intelligence, as well as conditions such as ADHD (Hauser et al. 1993).

Emotions

Because the body is flooded with sex hormones during adolescence, emotions are significantly affected during this time. It's similar to the upheaval we go through at perimenopause, when our hormones begin to ebb and flow in an erratic manner. (And, unfortunately, many of us go through this while our children are going through adolescence, making it an explosive situation!) Low thyroid function causes emotions to become exaggerated and unbalanced in children just as it does in adults, so unstable behavior may become the norm, especially emotional outbursts and rage, often coupled with paranoia and depression. This anguished emotional state is unfortunately a fertile breeding ground for development of substance abuse problems.

Recent research shows a connection between thyroid hormones and conditions such as bulimia and anorexia (Pritts and Susman 2003), which are rapidly increasing in the teenage population. Bipolar disorder (formerly called manic depression) is also becoming more and more common. Even schizophrenia is linked to low thyroid function. As you might guess, many of these adolescents respond beautifully to thyroid supplementation (Othman et al. 1994).

Lisa's Story

Lisa was a cheerful, outgoing tomboy throughout her childhood. She was good at team sports and enjoyed them, had lots of friends, and did well in school. But suddenly, when Lisa turned sixteen, her parents noticed changes in her behavior. She became sullen and uncommunicative, and when semester grades came out they realized that her grades were seriously slipping. She was moody and would go into a rage if questioned about homework, grades, or where she was going. She was also tired much of the time and insisted on quitting the soccer team, saying she didn't have the energy for sports as well as schoolwork.

Naturally, the first thing her parents suspected was drugs or alcohol because of the radical changes in her behavior. When they questioned her about this, she was indignant and offended and insisted that they were picking on her unfairly and that nothing was wrong. They were at a loss about what to do, as she refused to open up to them about what was bothering her. At about the same time, Lisa started to get severe acne and have very heavy menstrual periods that actually kept her home from school for a day or two almost every month. In a way, this was fortunate, as these physical symptoms became so distressing to Lisa that she agreed to go to her mother's ob-gyn for a checkup.

Lisa's mother had been seeing her doctor for low thyroid and other hormonal problems associated with perimenopause, and her doctor was an expert in the field of hormone imbalance. The first thing the doctor had Lisa do was complete an extensive health history. After reviewing this, the doctor explained that given Lisa's symptoms—emotional distress,

131

acne, menstrual irregularities, concentration problems, and fatigue—she was suspicious that Lisa was suffering from low thyroid function, just like her mother.

When her thyroid tests came back, the problem was clear. Lisa had low thyroid hormone levels, which explained all of her symptoms. Her doctor started her on supplemental thyroid hormones, and within the next few months most of her symptoms were resolved. Her acne cleared up, her menstrual cycles became lighter and less painful, and the changes in her behavior were amazing. Her cheerful, lively personality reappeared, and she noticed a huge difference in her ability to focus and study. And her parents were delighted; they felt they had gotten their daughter back.

EXERCISE: Children's Thyroid Symptom Evaluation

Read the following symptoms, decide on the level of severity or frequency of each sign or symptom in your child, and then circle the number that most accurately reflects how that statement applies to your child:

0 = None or never   1 = Mild or occasionally

2 = Moderate or often   3 = Severe or always

At the bottom of each page, total up the points circled, then carry these totals forward to the end of the evaluation to get a final score.

0	1	2	3	Multiple warts or moles
0	1	2	3	Bed-wetting after age six or seven
0	1	2	3	Teeth irregularities, such as late or irregular eruption, defective enamel, or numerous cavities
0	1	2	3	Nervousness or crying and screaming at the slightest provocation
0	1	2	3	Arms or legs short in proportion to the body
0	1	2	3	Difficulties with learning
0	1	2	3	Seemingly lazy or apathetic
0	1	2	3	Small pelvic bones and narrow hips
0	1	2	3	Pale toenail beds
0	1	2	3	Infantile jaundice, edema, umbilical hernia, or a larger than normal head
0	1	2	3	Straight, coarse hair
0	1	2	3	Swelling around the eyes

Page total: _____

0   1   2   3   Swollen lips

0   1   2   3   Swollen or larger than normal tongue, which can protrude from the mouth

0   1   2   3   Saddle nose, in which the bridge of the nose is depressed or flattened

0   1   2   3   Hoarse, soft voice

0   1   2   3   Overweight but not eating excessively

0   1   2   3   Cold feet and hands

0   1   2   3   Abnormally low or high birth weight

0   1   2   3   Recurrent ear infections or swimmer's ear

0   1   2   3   Much taller or shorter than peers

0   1   2   3   Chronic respiratory infections

0   1   2   3   Excessively quiet and withdrawn

0   1   2   3   Tired a lot of the time

0   1   2   3   Requires more sleep than most children

0   1   2   3   Dull, apathetic appearance with little expression

0   1   2   3   Broader than normal face

0   1   2   3   Noisy breathing

0   1   2   3   Cries for no apparent reason

0   1   2   3   Eyes more deep-set than usual

0   1   2   3   Started to crawl and walk late

0   1   2   3   Lacks normal coordination

0   1   2   3   Slow to start in the morning

0   1   2   3   Problems in school

0   1   2   3   Recurring swollen lymph glands

0   1   2   3   Menstrual irregularities such as heavy bleeding and cramping and irregular cycles

0   1   2   3   Lack of normal breast development

0   1   2   3   Highly emotional or given to temper tantrums

0   1   2   3   Short attention span

Page total: _____

0	1	2	3	Lack of self-confidence
0	1	2	3	Not comfortable socially
0	1	2	3	Can't sit quietly
0	1	2	3	Chronic tonsillitis
0	1	2	3	Precocious puberty (before age ten)
0	1	2	3	Delayed puberty (after age fifteen)
0	1	2	3	Mouth breathing or loud breathing
0	1	2	3	Anomalies genital development in male
0	1	2	3	Overdeveloped gums that extend down over the teeth and can appear swollen
0	1	2	3	Swollen female genitalia and poorly developed labia
0	1	2	3	Fat and flabby limbs
0	1	2	3	Excessive masturbation
0	1	2	3	Hands and feet plump and poorly shaped; short pyramidal fingers usually lying open due to defective muscle tone
0	1	2	3	Heavy and thick shoulders and hips
0	1	2	3	Scoliosis or lordosis (curvature of lower back)
0	1	2	3	Frequent nightmares
0	1	2	3	Diagnosed with ADHD or ADD
0	1	2	3	Flat feet
0	1	2	3	Chronic sprains
0	1	2	3	Kneecaps dislocated more than once
0	1	2	3	Digestive problems
0	1	2	3	Diagnosed with anemia
0	1	2	3	Diagnosed with bipolar disorder
0	1	2	3	Diagnosed with schizophrenia
0	1	2	3	Depression
0	1	2	3	Paranoia

Page total: _____

Total number of points: _____

Interpreting the Results

If your child's total points are between 12 and 18, he or she has signs of possible hypothyroidism. A score between 19 and 24 indicates that the condition is potentially more serious and your child could be experiencing significantly impaired thyroid function. With a score over 25 (or even one or two symptoms of particular severity, such as precocious puberty), your child should have a complete physical and a thyroid exam with lab tests, including measuring blood levels of free T3, free T4, TSH, and reverse T3, as well as thyroid antibodies if your doctor feels it's warranted. Since the thyroid is affected by the other endocrine glands, if your child is in puberty, it's also important to measure estrogen, progesterone, and testosterone in girls and testosterone in boys. It's advisable to measure cortisol levels as well, particularly if your child is sick a lot or has had a serious disease, such as mono.

WHAT'S NEXT?

Now that you've completed the Children's Thyroid Symptom Evaluation, you should have a much better understanding of your child's thyroid status. If your responses indicate potential hypothyroidism, schedule an appointment with your child's doctor as soon as possible so that you can have his or her thyroid examined and thyroid hormone levels tested. Armed with the results, you can start working on solutions. Take a copy of this completed evaluation with you to the appointment to give your child's doctor a complete picture of thyroid-related symptoms.

KEY POINTS

𝄞 Low levels of thyroid hormones can be devastating at any point in a pregnancy, as these hormones play a critical role in your baby's growth and development. Even a slight deficiency can result in low birth weight, lifelong small stature, and developmental abnormalities. Low thyroid function may be caused by hypothyroidism in the mother, insufficient function of the baby's thyroid gland, or iodine deficiency.

𝄞 In children, even relatively mild hypothyroidism can cause profound problems in physical and mental development, affecting them emotionally, cognitively, and physically.

𝄞 Hypothyroidism can cause completely opposite symptoms in different children. It can cause growth to be either accelerated or stunted, and may cause either hyperactivity or minimal and abnormally slow activity. Be on the lookout for symptoms at either end of the spectrum.

𝄞 Hypothyroidism can have heightened effects at puberty, including early or late onset of puberty and genital abnormalities, as well as menstrual problems in girls.

CHAPTER 11

Hyperthyroidism:
An Overactive Thyroid

Hyperthyroidism is essentially the opposite of hypothyroidism. Instead of producing too few thyroid hormones, in hyperthyroidism, the thyroid goes into overdrive and produces too much. At first glance, hyperthyroidism may sound attractive: If hypothyroidism means we get fat and tired, hyperthyroidism should mean thin and lively, right? Unfortunately, as so often occurs in life, too much of a good thing turns out to be a bad thing. An overabundance of thyroid hormones can damage your cells, particularly in your heart and bones, which increases your risk of heart damage and osteoporosis (Fadel et al. 2000).

Hyperthyroidism is much less common than hypothyroidism. The most common form is Graves' disease, and even it isn't very common, affecting only about 2 percent of women, usually during their thirties and forties (Reid and Wheeler 2005). With hyperthyroidism, the body's metabolism increases and affects how many calories you burn, how warm you feel, and how much you weigh. All of your cells respond to increases in thyroid hormones by increasing the rate at which they go about their business, causing you to feel hotter than those around you and also resulting in weight loss even though you may be eating more (although sometimes you can actually gain weight because of an increased appetite). You may be filled with energy at times, but it may be somewhat manic, and you'll usually experience fatigue at the end of the day but then have trouble sleeping. Your hands will tremble and you could develop an unusually forceful or irregular heartbeat (called palpitations). When the condition is very severe, you can become short of breath and experience chest pain. This constant bombardment with excessive amounts of thyroid hormones can make you easily upset and even irritable and also cause muscle weakness.

CAUSES OF HYPERTHYROIDISM

There are several different causes of hyperthyroidism: Graves' disease, thyroid nodules, thyroiditis, pituitary adenoma, and overdose of supplemental thyroid hormones. In addition, pregnancy can sometimes cause hyperthyroidism. (See "Pregnancy," in chapter 5, for full details.) It's important to determine the cause, since treatment varies depending on the underlying cause.

Graves' Disease

The most common cause of hyperthyroidism, accounting for about 95 percent of all cases, is a condition called Graves' disease, an autoimmune illness in which the immune system mistakenly directs an attack against healthy thyroid cells. These antibodies mimic the TSH that normally binds to receptors on the thyroid gland, stimulating it to produce more thyroid hormone (Braverman, Utiger, and Volpé 1991). The end result is that the thyroid cells continually produce and release thyroid hormones, overstimulating the body.

This disease causes a goiter, as the thyroid gland actually gets larger from making excessive amounts of thyroid hormones. This symptom can be confusing because the majority of thyroid goiters develop due to too little thyroid hormone production, rather than too much. The word "goiter" simply describes the oversized gland, not the cause of it. Graves' disease is more common in women in their thirties and forties, less common for those over age fifty, and tends to run in families.

Another symptom of Graves' disease is inflammation of the tissues around the eyes, causing swelling and eye irritation; it may also cause people to look like they are staring. A small number of people with Graves' disease have more severe eye problems, including severe inflammation, blurred or double vision, and bulging of the eyes (called exophthalmos). If these problems aren't treated, they can permanently damage the eyes and even cause blindness.

Nodules

Thyroid nodules are abnormal tumors or lumps in or on the thyroid gland. A single nodule, rather than the entire gland, can be responsible for excess hormone secretion. Thyroid nodules that produce excessive amounts of thyroid hormones are also sometimes called hot nodules or toxic nodular goiters. They're usually benign (noncancerous), but any lump, no matter what size, should be examined thoroughly to make sure it's not cancerous.

Thyroiditis

Thyroiditis, an inflammation of the thyroid gland, causes the thyroid to release excessive amounts of thyroid hormones. It is believed to be caused by a virus or pregnancy. The most common type is Hashimoto's disease, an autoimmune condition named after the doctor who discovered it.

In Hashimoto's thyroiditis, the immune cells known as lymphocytes invade the thyroid gland. This disrupts the sacs that store thyroid hormones, causing them to release the protein from which thyroid hormones are made, thyroglobulin, as well as thyroid peroxidase, an enzyme that aids in the production of T3 and T4. The released thyroglobulin and thyroid peroxidase irritate the body and cause antibodies to form, which damage the thyroid gland further and cause more sacs to rupture, spilling thyroid hormones into the bloodstream and overstimulating cells. This can result in symptoms of hyperthyroidism or fluctuation between symptoms of hypothyroidism and hyperthyroidism (Volpé 1990). In time, this process can destroy some or all of the thyroid, but it can also leave the thyroid gland completely normal (Durrant-Peatfield 2002).

Some types of thyroiditis can be painful, causing the front of the throat to be sore to the touch. Pain can also extend to the jaw or ear and can be confused with other conditions such as temporomandibular joint problems, ear infection, or strep throat.

Pituitary Adenoma

A benign tumor on the pituitary gland can cause independent production of many types of hormones, the most common being prolactin. In some cases, these growths produce an overabundance of TSH, resulting in excessive thyroid hormone production. Although described as benign because they're noncancerous, they can have serious adverse effects on the body.

Overdose of Supplemental Thyroid Hormones

Hyperthyroidism can also occur in people who take excessive doses of supplemental thyroid hormones. If you start taking thyroid hormones or increase your dose, you should keep the symptoms of excess thyroid activity described in chapter 3 in mind. If you develop any of these symptoms after starting thyroid hormone therapy, it's important to notify your doctor so you can adjust your dosage. You may also need to evaluate your adrenal function, as untreated adrenal fatigue can also cause symptoms of hyperthyroidism. (See "Treating Hypothyroidism When You Also Have Adrenal Fatigue," in chapter 7, for more information.)

LAB TESTS FOR HYPERTHYROIDISM

Lab tests for hyperthyroidism are the same as those for hypothyroidism: TSH, free T3, and free T4, as well as several thyroid antibody tests, including antibodies directed against thyroid peroxidase, thyroglobulin, and TSHr (thyroid-stimulating hormone receptors). All of these tests should be done first thing in the morning while fasting. A radioactive iodine uptake (RAIU) test is also often done to show areas of increased or decreased functioning of the thyroid by measuring the amount of radioactive iodine absorbed in the thyroid gland. The thyroid peroxidase antibodies (TPOAb) test is a blood test that measures levels of antibodies directed against thyroid peroxidase (TPO), an enzyme that aids in the production of T3 and T4. The thyroid-stimulating hormone receptor antibodies (TSHrAb) test is a blood test that looks for antibodies directed against thyroid-stimulating hormone receptors, which can cause Graves' disease. The thyroglobulin antibodies (TgAb) test is a blood test that measures thyroglobulin antibodies, which may also cause Graves' disease.

TREATMENT OF HYPERTHYROIDISM

Most treatments of hyperthyroidism are aimed at slowing the production of thyroid hormones. The most common treatments are medication, radioactive iodine treatment, surgery, and endocrine therapy.

Medication

There are various drugs available that either block the effects of excess thyroid hormones or make it difficult for the thyroid to use iodine to produce thyroid hormones. These medications are generally used as a temporary fix until something more permanent can be done. They're also prescribed for those who have a temporary form of hyperthyroidism.

Radioactive Iodine Treatment

Radioactive iodine treatment involves drinking radioactive iodine in order to destroy the thyroid's ability to make hormones. Iodine has an affinity for the thyroid gland and is actively attracted to it. When you add a radioactive substance to the iodine, much of this substance goes to the thyroid and damages or kills it.

Surgery

Surgery to remove all or part of the thyroid gland immediately reduces the levels of thyroid hormone in the body. However, it can result in facial nerve damage or paralysis of the vocal cords. Another possible side effect is damage to the parathyroids. Many people who have this surgery end up with hypothyroidism.

Endocrine Therapy

Some endocrinologists in the late 1800s and early 1900s believed that Graves' disease was caused by a genetic oversensitivity of the central nervous system, aggravated by a virus, other infection, or toxins, usually of an intestinal nature. This was thought to result in overstimulation of endocrine organs such as the adrenals, thymus, and thyroid, causing these glands to produce excessive amounts of hormones (Forchheimer 1906).

One of these early endocrinologists, Dr. Charles Sajous, believed that the best way to treat this condition was with thyroid hormone therapy. He said that the disease had three distinct phases, and that you had to be very cautious about using thyroid hormone therapy during the very early stage, as it would be like adding fuel to the fire. But in the second stage, where there was obvious hyperthyroid activity, thyroid supplementation had proven effective in calming this excessive activity down (Sajous 1903). Sajous believed that the overstimulation of the glands originated in the pituitary, and that adding thyroid hormones (and possibly cortisol) would calm the pituitary and stop it from continually stimulating other endocrine glands, thereby normalizing the feedback loops.

Obvious to say, this path is fraught with risk. It could exacerbate a hyperthyroid condition just as easily as resolve it. It's important to work with an experienced doctor to evaluate and treat hyperthyroidism with endocrine therapy, and ongoing monitoring is essential during treatment.

⫷ *Kristin's Story*

Kristin was thirteen years old when she started to develop symptoms of hyperthyroidism. She was very nervous and agitated, and she couldn't sleep. Her hands trembled, she had diarrhea and sweated constantly, and eventually her right eye started to bug out. Her parents took her to a pediatric endocrinologist, who ran tests that showed that she had elevated thyroid-stimulating hormone receptor (TSHr) antibodies. Kristin was diagnosed with Graves' disease.

Kristin's parents had numerous discussions with various doctors about the standard options for treating this condition, including drinking radioactive iodine or taking drugs to slow her thyroid function. But when they considered the side effects, such as liver damage, anemia, joint pain and swelling, and inflammation of the blood vessels, they decided to try another approach first.

Kristin had mononucleosis just prior to developing symptoms of hyperthyroidism, and this may have aggravated her central nervous system, ultimately resulting in overstimulation of her thyroid gland. Though it seemed counterintuitive, Kristin's doctor prescribed Armour Thyroid with the goal of normalizing the endocrine feedback loop responsible for her thyroid hyperactivity.

The result was amazing. Kristin's symptoms started to resolve almost immediately. The nervousness, trembling, and insomnia were the first symptoms to disappear. Everything else resolved over the next month except the exophthalmos condition of her eye, which took several months to return to normal. Subsequent lab tests showed no TSHr antibodies, so the treatment appeared to have resolved the autoimmune activity.

WHAT'S NEXT?

If you have some or all of the symptoms listed in this chapter, you may have hyperthyroidism. If so, schedule an appointment with your doctor as soon as possible to have your thyroid examined and your thyroid hormone levels tested to determine whether you have this condition. Carefully evaluate your options before starting any therapy that might have serious or long-term side effects.

KEY POINTS

- Symptoms of hyperthyroidism include heart palpitations or fast heart rate, overheating or heat intolerance, nervousness, insomnia, fatigue, irritability, trembling hands, weight loss, muscle weakness, warm and moist skin, and protruding, red, irritated eyes.

- Hyperthyroidism can damage your cells, particularly in your heart and bones, increasing your risk of heart damage and osteoporosis.

- Hyperthyroidism can be caused by Graves' disease, thyroid nodules, thyroiditis, pituitary adenoma, or an overdose of supplemental thyroid hormones.

- Methods of treating hyperthyroidism include medication, radioactive iodine treatment, surgery, or treatment of an underlying endocrine dysfunction possibly involving supplemental thyroid and adrenal hormones to normalize endocrine function.

Conclusion

I hope the information in this book has been helpful to you and that you're able to use it to restore your thyroid health and thereby enhance your health, happiness, and physical appearance for the rest of your life.

I know this process can be daunting, particularly if you've gone to your doctor and didn't get anywhere—or worse yet, if you suspect a thyroid problem but your doctor maintains your thyroid is fine and nothing more can be done for your symptoms. If this happens, remember, be confident, be educated, be assertive, and be positive. Stay focused on your goal and follow these simple steps:

Find the right doctor. Talk to your friends and local family members to find out if any of them have thyroid problems. If any of them do, ask them about the doctors they've seen and who they'd recommend. In particular, find out if any of them have seen doctors who have prescribed thyroid hormones, particularly Armour Thyroid. You may not need this specific type of therapy, but these doctors tend to be better versed in overall thyroid treatment and are open to the idea that treatments outside the conventional standard of care are sometimes necessary for optimal results. These doctors are also more likely to be aware that specialized tests may be necessary to get to the root cause of what's going on. And, most importantly, they generally understand that standard thyroid testing is just one tool and that it should be used in combination with a thorough evaluation of your symptoms to accurately diagnose thyroid problems.

Don't give up if your lab tests all come back normal. If you have many symptoms of hypothyroidism (or even just one or two obvious ones), you must persevere. You will need to be committed to see this through. Thyroid hormone resistance, elevated reverse T3, thyroid antibodies, thyroid hormone conversion problems, or problems with the pituitary or hypothalamus can all affect thyroid function. Doctors who aren't trained thyroid experts won't be aware of these conditions and probably won't be open to the idea that the usual lab tests don't tell the whole story. This is why finding the right doctor is so important.

Establish open lines of communication with your doctor. This is especially important when you start on thyroid hormone therapy. You may respond well to the first type of therapy your doctor puts you on, which in many cases will be a T4-only drug. But if you don't, be prepared to wage one last battle. Make sure your doctor understands how you're responding to the treatment. Collect specific, objective data to help your doctor understand what's going on. Avoid generalities like "I still don't feel well"; tell your doctor the specifics—the good and the bad. For instance, you may not be quite as tired as you were but still have chronic constipation, hair loss, and other symptoms of low thyroid function. Make sure your doctor knows all of this, as this scenario would indicate that the thyroid medication is affecting you positively, but it hasn't resolved all of your symptoms. In this case, it's likely that you need a different drug or a different dose. Don't settle for an inadequate or partial solution. Remember, you won't be settling for just thin hair or twenty extra pounds, you'll also be settling for a compromised immune system, neurological function, and endocrine system. This is *not* a good idea.

Interestingly, some the best general words of advice I've come across were from a book written by Arnold Lorand, MD, in 1910. He believed that achieving health and long life were completely within our grasp, and that disability and aging were due to a lack of information about how to keep the endocrine system healthy. He had thirteen basic tenants of health, which I believe are as valid today as they were a century ago:

1. Replace or reinforce the functions of endocrine organs affected by disease or age by using extracts of these organs from healthy animals, but *only* under the strict supervision of a doctor thoroughly familiar with the functions of these glands. (It's noteworthy that glandular extracts don't just provide supplemental hormones, they provide them in bioidentical forms.)

2. Spend as much time in the open air and sunshine as possible. Get plenty of exercise and breathe deeply and regularly while doing so.

3. Eat a diet consisting of meat once a day, eggs, cereals, green vegetables, fruit, and raw milk from healthy cows—and always chew thoroughly!

4. Take a bath daily, and every one to two weeks take a sauna.

5. Make sure to move your bowels daily.

6. Wear cotton, breathable underwear and low shoes, and keep your collar loose (don't compress that thyroid!).

7. Go to bed early and get up early.

8. Sleep in a very dark and quiet room with a window open (if possible). Don't sleep less than six hours or more than seven and a half hours for men and eight and a half hours for women.

9. Take one compete day of rest a week—without even reading or writing.

10. Avoid strong emotions and worries about things that have happened and can't be changed. Never say unpleasant things and avoid listening to them as well.

11. Get married (or in today's world, be in a committed relationship). Avoid excessive sexual activity but also avoid abstinence.

12. Use alcohol, tobacco, and caffeine very moderately (if at all).

13. Avoid overheated or poorly ventilated places.

Some of these will be easier to do than others. Who among us can take a full day off anymore? And while it's easy enough to recommend marriage, finding someone you actually want to commit to can be a different matter entirely. Of course most of us have seen those studies showing that people who own cats live much longer...possibly this will have to suffice.

I know I've given you an enormous amount of information to consider and digest. Some of it may seem daunting or even overwhelming at first, but don't despair. Go back to the chapters and sections that speak to your individual situation and reread them a few times. With repeated exposure, and with what you learn as you begin to study your symptoms, it will all start to make sense. Don't let the situation overwhelm you, just take it one step at a time—and always remember, your health and well-being are well worth this investment of your time and energy.

Good luck in your quest and let me know how you do!

In health,

Kathryn R. Simpson, MS
info@hormoneresource.com
www.hormoneresource.com

Resources

KATHRYN SIMPSON'S INFORMATION

Website: www.hormoneresource.com
Blog: http://mssolution.blogspot.com

DOCTOR REFERRALS

The following resources can help you locate physicians who may specialize in thyroid testing and treatment. Some are professional organizations with members who are more likely to specialize in hormones. After locating physicians in your area, you'll need to call them and talk to them or their staff to determine their level of expertise in thyroid testing and treatment.

American College for Advancement in Medicine (ACAM)
www.acamnet.org

American Academy of Anti-Aging Medicine (A4M)
www.worldhealth.net

American Holistic Medical Association (AHMA)
www.holisticmedicine.org

Health Professionals Directory
www.healthprofs.com/cam

Thyroid-Info.com
http://thyroid-info.com/topdrs/armour.htm

Compound Pharmacies
Compound pharmacies are good resources for finding doctors who specialize in treating thyroid disorders. These pharmacies make individualized bioidentical hormone preparations, so the pharmacy staff generally knows of local doctors prescribing such hormones. They will also know which doctors prescribe Armour Thyroid if you're interested in exploring this option. You can call the International Academy of Compounding Pharmacists (IACP) at (800) 927-4227 or see their website at www.iacprx.org to find a compounding pharmacy in your area.

Yellow Pages
If all else fails, look in the yellow pages under "physicians." Doctors who specialize in hormones often advertise themselves as holistic or complementary physicians.

References

Abraham, G. E., J. D. Flechas, and J. C. Hakala. 2002. Orthoiodosupplementation: Iodine sufficiency of the whole human body. *Original Internist* 9:30-41.

Agency for Toxic Substances and Disease Registry. 1999. Top 20 hazardous substances: From the CERCLA Priority List of Hazardous Substances for 2005. www.atsdr.cdc.gov/cxcx3.html. Accessed July 11, 2008.

Alvarez-Marfany, M., S. H. Roman, A. J. Drexler, C. Robertson, and A. Stagnaro-Green. 1994. Long-term prospective study of postpartum thyroid dysfunction in women with insulin dependent diabetes mellitus. *Journal of Clinical Endocrinology and Metabolism* 79(1):10-16.

American Association of Clinical Endocrinologists. 2007. Facts about common endocrine-related disorders. www.aace.com/meetings/ams/2007/Endodisfacts.php. Accessed May 23, 2008.

American Heart Association. 2008. Women and cardiovascular diseases: Statistics. Available at www.americanheart.org/presenter.jhtml?identifier=3000941. Accessed May 23, 2008.

Anasti, J. N., M. R. Flack, J. Froehlich, L. M. Nelson, and B. C. Nisula. 1995. A potential novel mechanism for precocious puberty in juvenile hypothyroidism. *Journal of Clinical Endocrinology and Metabolism* 80(1):276-279.

Ansquer, Y., A. Legrand, A. F. Bringuier, N. Vadrot, B. Lardeux, L. Mandelbrot, and G. Feldmann. 2005. Progesterone induces BRCA1 mRNA decrease, cell cycle alterations and apoptosis in the MCF7 breast cancer cell line. *Anticancer Research* 25(1A):243-248.

Arafah, B. M. 2001. Increased need for thyroxine in women with hypothyroidism during estrogen therapy. *The New England Journal of Medicine* 344(23):1743-1749.

Argov, Z., P. F. Renshaw, B. Boden, A. Winokur, and W. J. Bank. 1988. Effects of thyroid hormones on skeletal muscle bioenergetics: In vivo phosphorus-31 magnetic resonance spectroscopy study of humans and rats. *Journal of Clinical Investigation* 81(6):1695-1701.

Atroshi, I., C. Gummesson, E. Ornstein, R. Johnsson, and J. Ranstam. 2007. Carpal tunnel syndrome and keyboard use at work: A population-based study. *Arthritis and Rheumatism* 56(11):3620-3625.

Barker, L. F., R. G. Hoskins, and H. O. Mosenthal. 1922. *Endocrinology and Metabolism.* Vol. 1. New York: D. Appleton and Company.

Barnes, B. O., and L. Galton. 1976. *Hypothyroidism: The Unsuspected Illness.* New York: Harper & Row.

Bayraktar, M., and D. H. van Thiel. 1997. Abnormalities in measures of liver function and injury in thyroid disorders. *Hepatogastroenterology* 44(18):1614-1618.

Belviranli, M. 2006. The relation between reduced serum melatonin levels and zinc in rats with induced hypothyroidism. *Cell Biochemistry and Function* 26(1):19-23.

Blask, D. E., G. C. Brainard, R. T. Dauchy, J. P. Hanifin, L. K. Davidson, J. A. Krause, L. A. Sauer, M. A. Rivera-Bermudez, M. L. Dubocovich, S. A. Jasser, D. T. Lynch, M. D. Rollag, and F. Zalatan. 2005. Melatonin-depleted blood from premenopausal women exposed to light at night stimulates growth of human breast cancer xenografts in nude rats. *Cancer Research* 65(23):11174-11184.

Blizzard, R. M., D. Chee, and W. Davis. 1967. The incidence of adrenal and other antibodies in the sera of patients with idiopathic adrenal insufficiency (Addison's disease). *Clinical and Experimental Immunology* 2(1):19-30.

Bolk, N., T. Vissar, A. Kalsbeek, R. T. van Domburg, and A. Berghout. 2007. Effects of evening vs morning thyroxine ingestion on serum thyroid hormone profiles in hypothyroid patients. *Clinical Endocrinology* 66(1):43-48.

Braverman, L. E., R. D. Utiger, and R. Volpé. 1991. Grave's disease. In *Werner and Ingbar's The Thyroid: A Fundamental and Clinical Text*, ed. L. E. Braverman and R. D. Utiger. 6th edition. Philadelphia: Lippincott, Williams & Wilkins.

Brucker-Davis, F., M. C. Skarulis, A. Pikus, D. Ishizawar, M. A. Mastroianni, M. Koby, and B. D. Weintraub. 1996. Prevalence and mechanisms of hearing loss in patients with resistance to thyroid hormone. *Journal of Clinical Endocrinology and Metabolism* 81(8):2768-2772.

Bunevicius, R., G. Kazanavicius, R. Zalinkevicius, and A. J. Prange. 1999. Effects of thyroxine as compared with thyroxine plus triiodothyronine in patients with hypothyroidism. *New England Journal of Medicine* 340(6):424-429.

Castro, J. H., S. M. Genuth, and L. Klein. 1975. Comparative response to parathyroid hormone in hyperthyroidism and hypothyroidism. *Metabolism* 4(7):839-948.

Castro M. R., and H. Gharib. 2000. Thyroid nodules and cancer: When to wait and watch, when to refer. *Postgraduate Medicine* 107(1):113-124.

Cooper, J. G., K. Harboe, S. K. Frost, and Ø. Skadberg. 2005. Ciprofloxacin interacts with thyroid replacement therapy. *British Medical Journal* 330(7498):1002.

Datta, R. V., N. J. Petrelli, and J. Ramzy. 2006. Evaluation and management of incidentally discovered thyroid nodules. *Surgical Oncology* 15(1):33-42.

De Groot, L. J. 1999. Dangerous dogmas in medicine: The nonthyroidal illness syndrome. *Journal of Clinical Endocrinology and Metabolism* 84(1):151-164.

De Groot, L. J., G. Hennemann, and P. R. Larsen. 1984. *The Thyroid and Its Diseases.* New York: Churchill Livingston.

Diamond, J. 1985. *Life Energy.* New York: Paragon House.

Duncan, S. L. B. 1998. Disorders of Puberty. In *Gynaecology*, ed. R. Shaw, P. Soutter, and S. Stanton. Edinburgh: Churchill Livingstone.

Durrant-Peatfield, B. 2002. *The Great Thyroid Scandal and How to Survive It.* London: Barons Down.

Durrant-Peatfield, B. 2003. *Your Thyroid and How to Keep It Healthy.* London: Hammersmith Press.

Fadel, B. M., S. Ellahham, M. D. Ringel, J. Lindsay, L. Wartofsky, and K. D. Burman. 2000. Hyperthyroid heart disease. *Clinical Cardiology* 23(6):402-408.

Forchheimer, F. 1906. *The Prophylaxis and Treatment of Internal Diseases.* New York: Appleton Press.

Gardiner-Hill, H. 1937. Cretinism myxedema. *British Medical Journal* 1(3967):132-134.

Gawaii, H., Y. Friedrich, G. Dickstein, and Z. Friedman. 2003. Does hypothyroidism contribute to the etiology of primary open angle glaucoma or is it just a coincidence? [Article in Hebrew.] *Harefuah* 142(4):246-248.

Goglia, F., and P. DeLange. 2003. Non-nuclear actions of thyroid hormones: The case of T2. *Hot Thyroidology*, June.

Greenspan, F., and D. Gardner. 2000. *Basic and Clinical Endocrinology.* New York: McGraw Hill.

Haas, E., with B. Levin. 2006. *Staying Healthy with Nutrition.* Berkeley, CA: Celestial Arts.

Haddow, J. E., G. E. Palomaki, W. C. Allan, J. R. Williams, G. J. Knight, J. Gagnon, C. E. O'Heir, M. L. Mitchell, R. J. Hermos, S. E. Waisbren, J. D. Faix, and R. Z. Klein. 1999. Maternal thyroid deficiency during pregnancy and subsequent neuropsychological development of the child. *New England Journal of Medicine* 341(8):549-555.

Harrower, H. R. 1922. *Practical Organotherapy.* Glendale: The Harrower Laboratory.

Harrower, H. R. 1939. *An Endocrine Handbook.* Los Angeles: The Harrower Laboratory.

Hauser, P., A. J. Zametkin, P. Martinez, B. Vitiello, J. A. Matochik, A. J. Mixson, and B. D. Weintraub. 1993. Attention deficit-hyperactivity disorder in people with generalized resistance to thyroid hormone. *New England Journal of Medicine* 328(14):1038-1039.

Hertoghe, T. 2006. *The Hormone Handbook.* Surrey, UK: International Medical Books.

Hollowell, J. G., N. W. Staehling, W. H. Hannon, D. W. Flanders, E. W. Gunter, G. F. Maberly, L. E. Braverman, S. Pino, D. T. Miller, P. L. Garbe, D. M. DeLozier, and R. J. Jackson. 1998. Iodine nutrition in the United States. Trends and public health implications: Iodine excretion data from National Health and Nutrition Examination Surveys I and III (1971-1974 and 1988-1994). *Journal of Clinical Endocrinology and Metabolism* 83(10):3401-3408.

Hrynevych, I., H. D. Bendiuh, L. H. Iuhrinova, and T. N. Selezn'ova. 2002. Endocrine function of the thymus in experimental hypothyroidism. [Article in Ukrainian.] *Fiziologicheskii Zhurnal* 48(5):34-38.

Iervasi, G., A. Pingitore, P. Landi, M. Raciti, A. Ripoli, M. Scarlattini, A. L'Abbate, and L. Donato. 2003. Low-T3 syndrome: A strong prognostic predictor of death in patients with heart disease. *Circulation* 107(5):708-713.

Jabbour, S. A. 2003. Cutaneous manifestations of endocrine disorders: A guide for dermatologists. *American Journal of Clinical Dermatology* 4(5):315-331.

Jacobs-Kosmin, D. A., and R. J. B. DeHoratius. 2005. Musculoskeletal manifestations of endocrine disorders: Systemic disorders with rheumatic manifestations. *Current Opinion in Rheumatology* 17(1):64-69.

Janney, N. W. 1922. Hypothyroidism. In *Endocrinology and Metabolism,* ed. L. F. Barker, R. G. Hoskins, and H. O. Mosenthal. New York: D. Appleton and Company.

Jefferies, W. M. 1996. *Safe Uses of Cortisol.* Springfield, IL: C. C. Thomas.

Jiang, S., J. Lee, Z. Zhang, P. Inserra, D. Solkoff, and R. R. Watson. 1998. Dehydroepiandrosterone synergizes with antioxidant supplements for immune restoration in old as well as retrovirus-infected mice. *Journal of Nutritional Biochemistry* 9(7):362-369.

Kahaly, G. J., and W. H. Dillmann. 2005. Thyroid hormone action in the heart. *Endocrine Reviews* 1210(10):2003-2033.

Kendall, M. D. 1984. Have we underestimated the importance of the thymus in man? *Experientia* 40(11):1181-1185.

Klein, A. S., R. Lang, I. Eshel, Y. Sharabi, and J. Shoham. 1987. Modulation of immune response and tumor development in tumor-bearing mice treated by the thymic factor thymostimulin. *Cancer Research* 47(13):3351-3356.

LaFranchi, S. H., W. H. Murphey, T. P. Foley, P. R. Larsen, and N. R. M. Buist. 1979. Neonatal hypothyroidism detected by the Northwest Regional Screening Program. *Pediatrics* 63(2):180-191.

Lanni, A., A. Lombardi, M. Moreno, and F. Goglia. 1998. Effect of 3,5-di-iodo-L-thyronine on the mitochondrial energy-transduction apparatus. *Biochemical Journal* 330(1):521-526.

Lanni, A., M. Moreno, A. Lombardi, P. de Lange, E. Silvestri, M. Ragni, P. Farina, G. C. Baccari, P. Fallahi, A. Antonelli, and F. Goglia. 2005. 3,5-diiodo-L-thyronine powerfully reduces adiposity in rats by increasing the burning of fats. *FASEB Journal* 19(11):1552-1554.

Laughlin, G. A., and E. Barret-Connor. 2000. Sexual dimorphism in the influence of advanced aging on adrenal hormone levels: The Rancho Bernardo Study. *Journal of Clinical Endocrinology* 85(10):3561-3568.

Leckie, R. G., A. B. Buckner, and M. Bornemann. 1992. Seat belt-related thyroiditis documented with thyroid Tc-99m pertechnetate scans. *Clinical Nuclear Medicine* 17(11):859-860.

Lenzen, S., H. G. Joost, and A. Hasselblatt. 1976. Thyroid function and insulin secretion from the perfused pancreas in the rat. *Endocrinology* 99(1):125-129.

Li, L. 2003. The biochemistry and physiology of metallic fluoride: Action, mechanism and implications. *Critical Reviews in Oral Biology and Medicine* 14(2):100-114.

Liu, S., W. C. Willett, M. J. Stampfer, F. B. Hu, M. Franz, L. Sampson, C. H. Hennekens, and J. E. Manson. 2000. A prospective study of dietary glycemic load, carbohydrate intake, and risk of coronary heart disease in U.S. women. *American Journal of Clinical Nutrition* 71(6):1455-1461.

Lorand, A. 1910. *Old Age Deferred.* Philadelphia: F. A. Davis.

Lowe, J. C. 2000. *The Metabolic Treatment of Fibromyalgia.* Boulder, CO: McDowell Publishing.

Luecken, L. J., E. C. Suarez, C. M. Kuhn, J. C. Barefoot, J. A. Blumenthal, I. C. Siegler, and R. B. Williams. 1997. Stress in employed women: Impact of marital status and children at home on neurohormone output and home strain. *Psychosomatic Medicine* 59(4):352-359.

Madariaga, M. G., N. Gamarra, S. Dempsey, and C. P. Barsano. 2002. Thyroid polymyositis-lke syndrome in hypothyroidism: Review of cases reported over the past twenty-five years. *Thyroid* 12(4):331-336.

Malenchenko, A. F., E. P. Demidchik, and V. N. Tadeush. 1984. Content and distribution of iodine, chlorine and bromide in the normal and pathologically changed thyroid tissue. [Article in Russian.] *Meditsinskaia Radiologiia* 29(9):19-22.

Mann, D. 2002. Blind individuals have lower cancer risk: Melatonin link postulated. *International Journal of Humanities and Peace* 18:104.

Marqusee, E., J. A. Hill, and S. J. Mandel. 1997. Thyroiditis after pregnancy loss. *Journal of Clinical Endocrinology and Metabolism* 82(8):2455-2457.

Martin, S. 1995. Intestinal permeability. *BioMed Newsletter*, May, p. 11.

Mayo Foundation for Medical Education and Research. 2007. Depression and anxiety: Exercise eases symptoms. www.mayoclinic.com/health/depression-and-exercise/MH00043. Accessed May 23, 2008.

MedicineNet. 2008. Definition of standard of care. www.medterms.com/script/main/art.asp?article key=33263. Accessed May 23, 2008.

Moore, C. B., and T. D. Siopes. 2004. Spontaneous ovarian adenocarcinoma in the domestic turkey breeder hen: Effects of photoperiod and melatonin. *Neuroendocrinology Letters* 25(1-2):94-101.

Nash, J. W., C. Morrison, and W. L. Frankel. 2003. The utility of estrogen receptor and progesterone receptor immunohistochemistry in the distinction of metastatic breast carcinoma from other tumors in the liver. *Archives of Pathology and Laboratory Medicine* 127(12):1591-1595.

National Institute of Mental Health. 2008. The numbers count: Mental disorders in America. www.nimh.nih.gov/health/publications/the-numbers-count-mental-disorders-in-america.shtml. Accessed May 26, 2008.

Noren, J. G., and J. Alm. 1983. Congenital hypothyroidism and changes in the enamel of deciduous teeth. *Acta Paediatrica Scandinavica* 72(4):485-489.

Othman, S. S., K. A. Kadir, J. Hassan, G. K. Hong, B. B. Singh, and N. Raman. 1994. High prevalence of thyroid function test abnormalities in chronic schizophrenia. *Australian and New Zealand Journal of Psychiatry* 28(4):620-624.

Owen, P. J. D., and J. H. Lazarus. 2003. Subclinical hypothyroidism: The case for treatment. *Trends in Endocrinology and Metabolism* 14(6):257-261.

Pituitary Network Organization. 2007. Pituitary FAQs. www.pituitary.org/faq. Accessed May 31, 2008.

Pritts, S. D., and J. Susman. 2003. Diagnosis of eating disorders in primary care. *American Family Physician* 67(2):297-304.

Rabinowicz, T., D. E. Dean, J. M. Petetot, and G. M. de Courten-Myers. 1999. Gender differences in the human cerebral cortex: More neurons in males; more processes in females. *Journal of Child Neurology* 14(2):98-107.

Rajaratnam, S. A., and J. Arendt. 2001. Health in a 24-h society. *Lancet* 358(9286):999-1005.

Reid, J. R., and S. F. Wheeler. 2005. Hyperthyroidism: Diagnosis and treatment. *American Family Physician* 72(4):623-630.

Sainz, R. M., J. C. Mayo, D. X. Tan, L. León, L. Manchester, and R. J. Reiter. 2005. Melatonin reduces prostate cancer cell growth leading to neuroendocrine differentiation via a receptor and PKA independent mechanism. *Prostate* 63(1):29-43.

Sajous, C. E. M. 1903. *The Internal Secretions and the Principles of Medicine.* Philadelphia: F. A. Davis.

Sajous, C. E. M. 1914. *The Internal Secretions and the Principles of Medicine.* 6th edition. Philadelphia: F. A. Davis.

Sajous, C. E. M. 1922. *The Internal Secretions and the Principles of Medicine.* 10th edition. Philadelphia: F. A. Davis Company.

Sajous, C. E. M., and L. T. M. Sajous. 1930. *Sajous's Analytical Cyclopedia of Practical Medicine.* Vol. 8. Philadelphia: F. A. Davis Company.

Sandberg, P. O. 2008. Fine-needle aspiration of the thyroid gland: Its role in the investigation of thyroid autoimmunity. *Thyroid Science* 3(2):CLS1-2.

Schernhammer, E. S., F. Laden, F. E. Speizer, W. C. Willett, D. J. Hunter, I. Kawachi, C. S. Fuchs, and G. A. Colditz. 2003. Night-shift work and risk of colorectal cancer in the Nurses' Health Study. *Journal of the National Cancer Institute* 95(11):825-828.

Scobbo, R. R., T. W. VonDohlen, M. Hassan, and S. S. Islam. 2004. Serum TSH variability in normal individuals: The influence of time of sample collection. *West Virginia Medical Journal* 100(4):138-142.

Silva, J. E. 1995. Thyroid hormone control of thermogenesis and energy balance. *Thyroid* 5(6):481-492.

Simonides, W. S., C. van Hardeveld, and P. R. Larsen. 1992. Identification of sequences in the promoter of the fast isoform of sarcoplasmic reticulum Ca-ATPase required for transcriptional activation by thyroid hormone. *Thyroid* 2:S102.

Simpson, K. R., and D. E. Bredesen. 2006. *The Perimenopause and Menopause Workbook: A Comprehensive, Personalized Guide to Hormone Health.* Oakland, CA: New Harbinger Publications.

Singh, B., V. Chandran, H. K. Bandhu, B. R. Mittal, A. Bhattacharya, S. K. Jindal, and S. Varma. 2000. Impact of lead exposure on pituitary-thyroid axis in humans. *Biometals* 13(2):187-192.

Soma, K. K. 2006. Testosterone and aggression: Berthold, birds and beyond. *Journal of Neuroendocrinology* 18(7):543-551.

Spraul, M., E. Ravussin, A. M. Fontvieille, R. Rising, D. E. Larson, and E. A. Anderson. 1993. Reduced sympathetic nervous activity: A potential mechanism predisposing to body weight gain. *Journal of Clinical Investigation* 92(4):1730-1735.

Sterzl, I., J. Prochazkova, P. Hrda, P. Matucha, J. Bartova, and V. Stejskal. 2006. Removal of dental amalgam decreases anti-TPO and anti-Tg autoantibodies in patients with autoimmune thyroiditis. *Neuro Endocrinology Letters* 27(suppl. 1):25-30.

Stokkan, K. A., and R. J. Reiter. 1994. Melatonin rhythms in Arctic urban residents. *Journal of Pineal Research* 16(1):33-36.

Stratmoen, J. 2005. High incidence of hypopituitarism among traumatic brain injury patients. *Neurology Today* 5(3):84-85.

Substance Abuse and Mental Health Services Administration. 2005. Depression among adults. *The National Survey on Drug Use and Health Report*, November 18. www.oas.samhsa.gov/2k5/depression/depression.htm. Accessed May 26, 2008.

Tan, E. K., S. C. Ho, P. Eng, L. M. Loh, L. Koh, S. Y. Lum, M. L. Teoh, Y. Yih, and D. Khoo. 2005. Restless legs symptoms in thyroid disorders. *Parkinsonism and Related Disorders* 10(3):149-151.

Trainin, N., and M. Linker-Israeli. 1976. Restoration of immunologic reactivity of thymectomized mice by calf thymus extracts. *Cancer Research* 27(2):309-313.

Vijayalaxmi, C. R. Thomas, R. J. Reiter, and T. S. Herman. 2002. Melatonin: From basic research to cancer treatment clinics. *Journal of Clinical Oncology* 20(10):2575-2601.

Van Vollenhoven, R. F. V., E. G. Engleman, and J. L. McGuire. 1994. An open study of dehydroepiandrosterone in systemic lupus erythematosus. *Arthritis and Rheumatism* 37(9):1305-1310.

Vincent, S. 1912. *Internal Secretion and the Ductless Glands.* London: Edward Arnold.

Volpé, R. 1990. Immunology of human thyroid disease. In *Autoimmunity and Endocrine Disease.* Boca Raton, FL: CRC Press.

Waller, D. K., J. L. Anderson, F. Lorey, and G. C. Cunningham. 2000. Risk factors for congenital hypothyroidism: An investigation of infant's birth weight, ethnicity, and gender in California, 1990-1998. *Teratology* 62(1):36-41.

Wartofsky, L., and R. A. Dickey. 2005. Controversy in clinical endocrinology: The evidence for a narrower thyrotropin reference range is compelling. *The Journal of Clinical Endocrinology and Metabolism* 90(9):5483-5488.

Wikland, B. 2008a. Redefining hypothyroidism: A paradigm shift. *Thyroid Science* 3(1):E1.

Wikland, B. 2008b. What is optimal treatment of hypothyroidism? A matter of clinical common sense. *Thyroid Science* 3(1):H1.

Kathryn R. Simpson, MS, was an executive in the biotech industry when she was diagnosed with multiple sclerosis. Research led her to discover that her symptoms were caused by multiple hormonal deficiencies including low thyroid, adrenal, and sex hormone levels. She resolved all of her debilitating symptoms with bio-identical hormone supplementation. Simpson founded a specialty hormone clinic, the Simpson Foundation, to treat hormone imbalance and diseases such as multiple sclerosis, lupus, and fibromyalgia. Today, the Simpson Foundation is dedicated to endocrine research and education. Simpson is author of *The Perimenopause and Menopause Workbook* and *The MS Solution*. She lives in Santa Ynez, CA.

Foreword writer **Thierry Hertoghe, MD,** is a fourth-generation endocrinology expert. His great-grandfather, grandfather, and father were pioneers in early endocrinology and thyroid research. Hertoghe is author of *The Hormone Solution* and *The Hormone Handbook*.

Other Books by Kathryn R. Simpson

The Perimenopause and Menopause Workbook: A Comprehensive, Personalized Guide to Hormone Health for Women (with Dale E. Bredesen). Oakland, CA: New Harbinger Publications, 2006.

The MS Solution: How I Solved the Puzzle of My Multiple Sclerosis. Santa Ynez, CA: Los Olivos Publishing, 2008.

Index

causes of hypothyroidism, 55-68; adrenal complications, 67; antibodies, 60;
conversion problems, 66; environmental toxins, 62-63; foreign invaders, 60-61; genetics, 64-65; hypothalamus or pituitary problems, 59; iodine deficiency, 63; medications, 62; ovarian function changes, 55-57; physical injury, 61-62; pregnancy, 57-59; thyroid hormone resistance, 66-67
central hypothyroidism, 59
chemicals, toxic, 100-101
childbirth, 53
childhood thyroid dysfunction, 125-136; early childhood and, 127-129; evaluating symptoms of, 132-135; gestation and, 126; infancy and, 126-127; puberty and, 129-132
cholesterol, 47, 48
chronic inflammatory diseases, 111
ciprofloxacin, 88
circadian rhythm, 17
cognitive ability, 45, 130-131
complex carbohydrates, 23, 94, 95
compound pharmacies, 148
constipation, 47
conversion problems, 66
Cooper, Astley, 6
cortisol, 106-107; lifestyle choices and, 121-123; production pattern for, 107-108; stress and, 22, 109-110; supplemental, 120; symptoms of excess, 109; testing levels of, 118
cretinism, 125
Cushing's disease, 119

D

dehydration, 111
dental problems, 41
depression, 44-45
DHEA, 107; cortisol levels and, 109; immune function and, 111; supplemental, 121
DHEA sulfate (DHEA-S) test, 119
diabetes, 23
diarrhea, 90
diet/nutrition, 94-98; adrenal function and, 122; balancing foods in, 94-96; basic guidelines for, 96-97; fad diets and, 95; food additives and, 101; importance of iodine in, 97; nutritional supplements and, 97, 98, 122; thyroid function and, 94-98
digestion problems, 47, 102
digestive enzymes, 23, 47
diiodotyrosine (T2), 10-11
disease: hypothyroidism and, 8-9, 51-52. *See also* immune system

dizziness, 49
doctors: choosing, 70, 143; communicating with, 144; resources for locating, 147-148
drugs. *See* medications
Durrant-Peatfield, Barry, 61, 80, 109

E

ear infections, 42
early childhood, 127-129
edema, 40, 46
elimination problems, 47
emotions: adolescent development and, 131; hypothyroidism and, 44-45
endocrine system, 15-26; adrenal glands, 22-23; checks and balances in, 16; function of, 15-16; hypothalamus, 18-19; pancreas, 23; parathyroid glands, 21; pineal gland, 16-18; pituitary gland, 19; reproductive glands, 24-25; thymus, 21-22; thyroid gland, 19-21
endocrine therapy, 141
energy level, 51
environmental toxins, 62-63
estrogen, 24-25; DHEA supplements and, 121; insulin resistance and, 23; progesterone and, 24-25, 56-57; thyroid hormones and, 24, 88, 91
estrogen dominance, 24-25
evaluating thyroid function. *See* assessment of thyroid function
exercise: adrenal function and, 121-122; thyroid function and, 99
eyebrows, 40
eyesight problems, 49

F

facial features, 40
fad diets, 95
family health history, 64-65
fats, dietary, 94
female hormones, 24-25, 52-53
fetal development., 126
fight-or-flight hormones, 106
fingernails, 41
fludrocortisone, 120
fluid retention, 46
fluoxetine, 45, 89
follicle-stimulating hormone (FSH), 19
food: additives/alteration, 101; allergies, 101-102. *See also* diet/nutrition
foot and leg problems, 41-42
free T3 and T4 tests, 74
fungal infections, 60

liver function, 48
Lorand, Arnold, 144
low blood pressure, 46, 111, 117
luteinizing hormone (LH), 19

M

medications: antibiotic, 8; antidepressant, 44-45, 89; hyperthyroidism and, 140; hypothyroidism and, 62; interactions between, 88-89; thyroid, 82-83
melatonin, 17-18
memory, 45
menopause, 24
menstrual cycle, 52-53, 56-57
mercury, 100
metabolic damage, 101-103
metals, toxic, 99-100
mind and emotions, 44-45
mineral supplements, 88, 97, 98, 122
miscarriages, 53
mitochondria, 20, 102
mobility problems, 48-49
monoiodotyrosine (T1), 10-11
mouth problems, 41
muscle problems, 43
myxedema, 37, 40, 46

N

needle biopsy, 61
negative feedback system, 16
nerve function, 48
nervous system, 15
night shift workers, 18
noradrenaline, 106
nutrition. *See* diet/nutrition

O

ovarian cancer, 18
ovarian function, 55-57
ovaries, 24, 52, 55
overactive thyroid. *See* hyperthyroidism
ovulation, 56-57
oxytocin, 19

P

pain, 51
pancreas, 23
parathyroid glands, 21
perimenopause, 24, 52, 55

Perimenopause and Menopause Workbook, The (Simpson and Bredesen), 28, 56
phosphatidylserine, 122-123
physical activity, 99
physical appearance, 39-44
physical growth, 130
physical injury, 61-62
pinch test for myxedema, 37
pineal gland, 16-18
pituitary adenoma, 139
pituitary gland, 10, 19, 59, 71, 139
pollutants, 100-101
posture problems, 42
pregnancy, 53, 57-59
pregnenolone, 109, 123
probiotics, 102
professional organizations, 147-148
progesterone, 24-25, 56-57
prolactin, 19
protein, 94
psychological health, 44-45
puberty, 52, 129-132; cognitive function in, 130-131; emotions in, 131; physical growth in, 130; sexual development in, 129-130
pulse rate, 47
pupil contraction test, 117

R

radioactive iodine, 62, 140
refined carbohydrates, 23, 95-96
reproductive glands, 24-25
resources, information, 147-148
restless legs syndrome (RLS), 48
reverse T3 (rT3): conversion problems, 66; testing for, 74-75

S

Sajous, Charles, 8, 141
saliva testing, 118
salt, 37, 63, 97, 110
seasonal affective disorder (SAD), 17
secondary hypothyroidism, 59
serotonin, 17
sexual development, 129-130
sexual function, 53
skin problems, 40
sleep: hypothyroidism and, 49; importance of getting, 98; melatonin production and, 18
social isolation, 45
soy products, 96

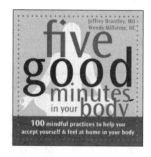
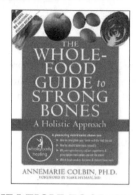
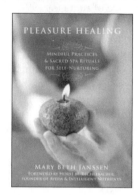
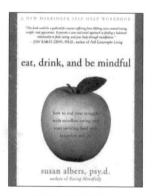
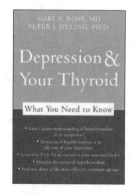
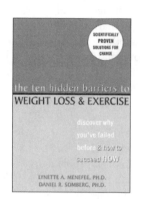